# Answers in the Dark

## Grief, Sleep and How Dreams Can Help You Heal

# Answers in the Dark

## Grief, Sleep and How Dreams Can Help You Heal

### Delphi Ellis

BOOKS

Winchester, UK
Washington, USA

JOHN HUNT PUBLISHING

First published by O-Books, 2022
O-Books is an imprint of John Hunt Publishing Ltd., 3 East St., Alresford,
Hampshire SO24 9EE, UK
office@jhpbooks.com
www.johnhuntpublishing.com
www.o-books.com

For distributor details and how to order please visit the 'Ordering' section on our website.

ISBN: 978 1 78535 651 3
978 1 78535 652 0 (ebook)
Library of Congress Control Number: 2021930251

A CIP catalogue record for this book is available from the British Library.

Design: Stuart Davies

UK: Printed and bound by CPI Group (UK) Ltd, Croydon, CR0 4YY
Printed in North America by CPI GPS partners

We operate a distinctive and ethical publishing philosophy in
all areas of our business, from our global network of authors to
production and worldwide distribution.

# Contents

# Acknowledgements

When writing this expression of thanks, I realised just how many people – and specifically how we met – had so much to do with its creation. It was made possible through a lifetime of experiences so far, including the privilege of working alongside people who have shared with me their journeys to recovery. Their stories, if included here, are done in such a way their identity is protected; my wholehearted thanks go to all of them, past and present. Thanks also go to my first work mentor, Dave, whose encouragement for reaching my potential enabled the path of helping others that I'm on now. To my tutor Chris, for his wisdom in exploring mindfulness in therapeutic work all those years ago. To Kylie Holmes, an author herself, who always believed I could write this book. To Bhante, in metta for his teachings and insight, available on speed dial (what he calls "Dial a Monk"), and always with a smile. To my mum, who tells me, "Everything that is, isn't and everything that isn't, is," for sharing her insights on dreams which lit my passion for the subject. My dad, for the love he was able to give; his death literally changed the course of my life. To my clinical supervisors over the years, especially Gareth and Jackie, for helping me work effectively in service to others. To Jim for, well, you'll see why. To Dean for his unwavering friendship. To Steve for making sure I was fed and watered whilst writing, and on many occasions where I'd ask, "What's the word for...?" And my children, friends, family and loved ones, for their continued support and patience, in making this book (long in the writing!) possible.

To my children
You are my dreams come true.

**dream**
driːm/
noun
noun: dream; plural noun: dreams
1. "a series of thoughts, images, and sensations occurring in a person's mind during sleep".

**sleep**
sliːp/
noun: sleep
1. "a condition of body and mind which typically recurs for several hours every night".

Or not, as the case may be...

# Preface

As I'm writing this preface, we are slowly navigating our way out of the first wave of the COVID-19 pandemic. This book, whilst nearly 10 years in the planning, couldn't have found a more relevant time to be published. People can't sleep and if they can, they're having the wildest, most vivid dreams.

Since the Coronavirus outbreak, according to the Lyon Neuroscience Research Centre,[1] dream recall increased 35% among participants in their research study. One reason may be that instead of getting up at the crack of dawn for our early morning commute, we might be staying in bed a little later, and by doing so, dreaming a bit longer. So this is normal.

It makes perfect sense if you've been remembering more dreams since COVID-19 kicked off, and if they're more negative than usual. Our lives have changed dramatically. Bizarre or troubling dreams are to be expected; they are *not* a sign there is something inherently wrong with you.

Yet we worry about dreams, especially when we think they make us look a bit weird. The reason for this, as I will expand on later, is largely steeped in centuries of myths and legends, and questionable theories from people like that man with the beard you might have heard of called Freud. (I say it like this, because whenever I mention him, someone usually says, "Is he the one with the beard?")

If nothing else, this book aims to reassure you, that your dreams are okay even if *you're* not feeling okay right now. In fact, your dreams may be able to help.

COVID-19 has highlighted many things. Whilst it has been busy causing disruption, uncertainty, heartache and chaos, the outbreak reminded us, in the words of Life. Death. Whatever. (@lifedeathwhat), that grief doesn't just belong to death.

It can be the loss associated with the holiday you *really*

needed but had to cancel. It might be in the work you can't do because you've been furloughed or made redundant. Or in literally having to distance yourself from the people you love. The absence of connection has been palpable. Loneliness has touched all parts of society. And frankly, we've all been hug deficient; that's bound to take its toll.

Then there's the tiredness.

We've discovered Zoom fatigue, where online meetings require extraordinary levels of concentration, alongside decision fatigue that comes from trying to do our best to run a home doubling as a workspace; the boundaries between work and home life are blurred more than ever.

For those of us familiar with working from home, it's been *far* from normal; we're not working under ordinary conditions. We're trying to work, home school and/or care for sick relatives in the midst of a worldwide crisis. Just when we think we've adapted to the "new normal", the rules change again.

No wonder so many of us are exhausted, and maybe even a bit scared. You'd think we would just flop in to bed at night, and pass out within minutes, from the mental drain and sheer overwhelm of it all... and yet we don't.

This is because vivid dream recall and a poor night's sleep are not unique to a worldwide pandemic. As I'll explain in this book, the impact of everyday life, including all that comes with it, and the loss of cultural conversations around death and dying, has affected our ability to rest and relax.

I will be expanding beyond the relationship between sleep and mental health, by recognising how the losses we face throughout our lives, as we navigate being human, can remain unresolved and go underground until they find their way in to the light – sometimes in the guise of what we dream.

The book provides tools like the Sleep Cycle Repair Kit to discuss basic tips, and then a wider set of activities to try once you're in bed, when you're inevitably staring up at the ceiling.

If you're being woken up by nightmares or weird dreams, I'll cover that too.

The book is split in to three parts: Part I busts some myths about sleep and dreams in general, and why I think grief has a role to play in this. Part II focuses on how to sleep better, based on what I've learned and people find helpful. Part III specifically explores dreams and why we have them. It all knits together, but you can dip in and out of it if you prefer.

## What this book isn't

*Answers in the Dark* is not a dream dictionary nor is it a complete catalogue of different types of dreams, for one simple reason: what you dream is unique to you, and only you have the key that unlocks what's inside. The reason the media call me a "Dream Expert" is not because I have all the answers to what your dream means, but because I've been researching this topic since long before I went on the telly.

Whilst people have tried for centuries to tell us what dreams mean, I have always felt analysis should be a personal exploration for the dreamer (alongside, if they choose, a friend or therapist). However, it is not, and never will be, a "one-size-fits-all" philosophy. It is not for anyone to tell you definitively what your dream means, me included. Because, it's *your* dream.

In the same way, I've explored the nature of sleep, what seems to get in the way and what can help, recognising that everyone is different. I include research where I think it's relevant, but not in a wordy, jargon-y, academic way because there's loads of books like that if you prefer them. Rather than include references to the published works, I've used links to the plain-English articles which where possible contain the publications, so that you can choose which you prefer to read.

Where I've spoken about specific people and their experiences, I've changed their name and some of the details of their story in order to protect their identity.

What this book also does, is build on the themes, experiences, myths and frequently asked questions I've worked with over decades. It gives you tools to help with what might be keeping you awake at night, and how to explore your own dreams to build a picture of what they might be trying to say.

As sciences, sleep and dream research are still relatively new, so theories around how to sleep and why we dream are changing all the time. As Adam Rutherford explains of science, in his important book *How to Argue With a Racist*:

*Scientists disagree all the time about the significance of results, or the techniques deployed in their analyses. It is perfectly possible for a paper in a reputable journal to be flawed, or even wrong.*

My point is, what I've written today might be out of date tomorrow, so take what you feel will help your current situation and leave the rest.

The book is written from a more client-focused model that's holistic and focused on your well-being, rather than a medical one. It's particularly for people with mild to moderate mental health considerations, like stress, depression and anxiety, in mind.

Working as a mental health professional, I know that telling you to cheer up or look on the bright side (which I would never say) is the last thing you probably need to hear right now.

I know it's not a simple case to "snap out of it", from whatever is stopping you sleeping. I'm not a person who might suggest that the reason you can't sleep is because you're flawed in some way – I don't believe you are. I won't tell you that you must be doing something wrong; I know you've probably tried *everything* to sleep – and dream – better.

This book does talk, usually in a light-hearted way, about making friends with the dark because, generally speaking, we fear it more than we need. I believe time spent at night –

both awake and asleep – can provide fascinating insights and wisdom, once you know how, so you might want to keep a journal throughout this process.

I take seriously, though, that for many people night-time has not always been a safe place. If you have been impacted by trauma, or a life-changing situation which has a severe or enduring impact on your mental health, then please create safe spaces for yourself if you continue reading this book, and make room for plenty of self-care. Speak to your doctor or healthcare team before you try the activities suggested throughout, and have people nearby that you trust, to support you if needed. The Samaritans are available as a listening service in the UK 24/7 on 116 123 and you'll see me repeat that number a lot. There is also a list of links to various agencies at the back which may help.

What I aim to do is reassure you that how you feel is valid, that you're not alone and help is available; that by picking up this book you have already taken a significant step. Here begins a fascinating journey of discovery, and potentially transformative personal development.

# Introduction: Help for a Sleepless Society

*To sleep, perchance to dream*
~ *Hamlet*

Sleep could be described as something of a paradox in the 21st Century. It's essential, but it's inconvenient. We want it, but we can't always achieve it. It should be a friend, but can feel like the enemy. It's promising, but can be something of a disappointment. It's like buying a scratch card: you can see the potential of trying, but then wonder why you bothered.

To me, the bedroom is the night-time equivalent of Schrödinger's Cat experiment: an intriguing four-sided container where the outcome remains a mystery until you dive in. You don't really know the result until you go to bed and, although you always set out with good intentions to sleep well, ultimately you either will or you won't. It could end in relief, or feel like an absolute disaster.

Depending on how well you've been sleeping lately, you'll already have a sense as to whether or not you're going to get some sleep tonight. Feeling tired and exhausted, you may hope that tonight will be the night your head hits the pillow and you'll pass out into a gorgeous dream land. If you do manage to doze off it may seem only a couple of hours later, you find yourself awake until the early hours, wondering what on earth went wrong.

If you've not been sleeping well for a while, at best you might approach bedtime with a vague hope you'll eventually nod off, but with perhaps a sense of quiet resignation that it won't necessarily be the refreshing sleep you need. At worst, you may be dreading going to your bed, for fear of thoughts, feelings and bad dreams you worry the dark may bring.

To paraphrase Hamlet, sleep is either to be or not to be. And if it's not to be, it can feel like a tragedy waiting to happen.

In the UK, we are a nation of poor sleepers,[2] and insomnia – essentially, trouble falling asleep or staying asleep – is a problem on a global scale. According to one study by insurance company Aviva, 37 per cent of adults in Britain (compared to 31 per cent in the US and Canada) say they don't sleep enough, with more than two in five so worn out they had no energy to exercise. Twenty per cent of the global population suffer from insomnia.[3]

According to the Big Sleep Report (Meadows, 2017), only 1 per cent of British people wake up feeling refreshed. Even those who reach the holy grail of eight hours every night (which, in all the years I've been talking about this, is rare), they will admit when they wake up, they feel they could still do with a few more hours kip.

Generally speaking, people around the world are shattered.

Tired but wired.

Running on empty.

Sleep deprived, but wide awake.

Sound familiar?

Welcome to our Sleepless Society.[4]

Various health agencies aren't shy in telling us the impact sleepless nights are having. Reports from the World Health Organization[5] quote that lack of sleep can make us more susceptible to minor ailments like coughs and colds, and major diseases like heart disease, cancer and Alzheimer's.

Research also suggests that missing out on the process of dreaming (through lack of sleep) can take its toll on our mental health and memory.[6] But I'm not going to keep on, because I genuinely don't know anyone who wants to hear all this.

You know how you feel when you've had a rough night. You know how hard it is to concentrate and stay focused when you're tired. You understand how your mood is affected, and how you struggle to find motivation, because you're living it every day. Me telling you how bad it is, or what researchers say will happen if you don't get some decent sleep soon, isn't useful.

What you probably want to know is how to make it better.

It's usually then that you might go online or pick up the latest magazine with a "special edition on sleep" to find out the latest top tips. (I'm saying this, because in the past I've done it.)

So we search the Internet, which invariably offers up the same advice around what's commonly known as Sleep Hygiene. This is not whether or not you're washing your armpits before bed; it's the habits we have during the day that either help you or stop you sleeping at night.

It usually includes advice about reducing your caffeine intake and switching off your phone at some reasonable point during the evening. If you've ever approached work about this (especially your Occupational Health department or seen the HR/well-being newsletter that goes out around World Sleep Day in March) they will usually talk about what you should be doing different.

Whilst having good habits in the day can definitely help (see the Sleep Cycle Repair Kit later), sleep hygiene is just one part of achieving better sleep and dreams. And people are a bit fed up of hearing about it.

Almost everyone I teach or talk with knows all about sleep hygiene. They get how important sleep is. They know they can't outsource sleep to someone else, neither can they bypass it (at least not for any reasonable length of time). They understand cutting down on coffee is good, and lavender is nature's remedy for rest and relaxation, because they've tried it – *all* of it – and they *still* can't sleep.

By the time people talk to me, they've usually reached the conclusion there must be something fundamentally wrong with them, because they've tried every trick in the book (except maybe the book you're reading now).

They've switched to decaf.

They're having a warm bath before bed.

They're turning off their phone, and have classical music, like Bach's *Goldberg Aria*, playing in the background.

They may even have gone to their doctor for medication to help.

Don't get me wrong, sleep hygiene matters. Whether it's the natural progression of the menopause, or medical conditions which cause physical pain that impact our ability to rest, our daytime habits can still affect night-time rest. But counting sheep and having a warm milky drink before bed isn't always the answer. Nor does it get to the *actual* cause.

When you genuinely believe you've done your best, you would understandably be left feeling hopeless and confused. And then, because you've tried *everything*, and still can't sleep, you might think it must be an inherent flaw. But, as I'll come on to explain, I don't believe that's the case.

So why is good quality, refreshing sleep escaping the population, and was even before we had a global health emergency? How is it that when you've tried all the things that health agencies, colleagues and medical professionals recommend, it just doesn't work? The answers, I believe, might be in the dark itself.

When sleep has escaped you for so long, it's not necessarily because of something you're consciously *doing*, but because of a situation that may be resting underneath awareness.

It might be the emotions around a past hurt, like a relationship breakdown or bereavement, have gone underground and are trying to find their way out. (The etymology of the word "depressed" means something which has been "pushed down".) It might be something that's nagging at your thoughts about work or home, but you can't make sense of right now.

This is my definition of "Situational Insomnia": it's not always what you do that stops you sleeping, but what has happened – or is happening – *to* you.

## About the Science

Although sleep in itself is not something new, we've only been scratching the surface of its science for about 100 years. For the most part, it all started around the invention of the electroencephalograph (or EEG).

In 1924, Hans Berger first used the EEG to record brain waves. Then in 1953 Eugene Aserinsky and Nathaniel Kleitman were able to use it to define what they called Rapid Eye Movement (REM), the stage of sleep most commonly associated with dreaming.

Aserinsky and Kleitman are generally considered to be the founders of modern sleep research, although it was William Dement, named "The Father of Sleep Medicine", who detailed the sleep phases, conducting some of the earliest studies around the dreaming stage. (It was noted that when Dement died, in June 2020 aged 91, he did so in his sleep.[7])

Today, the study of sleep continues and opinions are changing *all* the time. This means that the guidance sleep experts used to give years ago – such as telling you to get up if you wake up, may not be the only path to take now. (I'll expand on this in Part II.)

One of the reasons *Answers in the Dark* has taken me so long to write is because every time "ground-breaking" research claimed to have discovered the secrets of sleep and dreams – and scientists would promote a new "one-size-fits-all" methodology – I would consider including it in this book, and then someone would come along and say it's *just not that simple*. (Okay, I will admit, I am usually one of those saying that.)

Everyone is different, and you can't put people in boxes like that. When I realised that writing a book on this topic, in an ever-changing landscape, is (as my mum would say) like trying to pin gravy to the wall, I made the decision to focus less on the medical, academic approach of problem solving, and more on what I know best: working with people. Humans are not simply problems that need fixing. We are all just doing the best we can, with what we have from where we are.

I have the utmost respect for researchers in this arena, who painstakingly investigate with good intentions how we sleep and why we dream; they literally dedicate their lives to this work, as Dement did. But when the whole topic became so studious that people tell me the prescribed solutions (like sleep hygiene) aren't working, or they've been labelled "non-compliant" or "beyond help" because they don't want to take a drug to feel better, I decided it's time to talk about it the way I teach it.

In the last two decades, I have taught and worked with hundreds of people, and what I offer is simply food for thought.

While the science of sleep may still be evolving, the foundations of what I've discovered to be the causes of poor sleep – and what helps improve it – have fundamentally remained the same. Some researchers and academics may not like the way I'm delivering it, but this book isn't for them; it's for those who no matter what they do, night-time has become a nightmare.

In the next chapter, Faulty Winks, I explain my background, and how dreams and sleep became such an important part of what I do. From there, I'll expand on why I think you might find some of the answers in the dark.

So, in the style of a good old-fashioned bedtime story, are you ready?

Then, I'll begin.

*Nod to Sleep History:*

*In 1741, Johann Sebastian Bach wrote the* Goldberg Variations, *to be played by his associate Johann Gottlieb Goldberg for Count Kaiserling, a former Russian Ambassador.*

*Goldberg, who played the clavier, reportedly shared a house with Kaiserling, who suffered with insomnia at the time. The variations were written for the harpsichord, the tone of which some people now believe can help ease insomnia.*

*In 2005, the* Journal of Advanced Nursing *reported that listening to calming music before bed could help you sleep better,*[8] *citing that a tempo of 60-80 beats per minute, found in some classical music and pieces of jazz, has been shown to have a soporific effect. Other researchers noted that the opening* Aria *of the* Goldberg Variations *could be played at a tempo of 60-80 beats per minute; so even before sleep science was a thing, Bach was literally on the right track.*

# Part I

# Faulty Winks

*Lack of sleep is only bad if you have to drive, or think, or talk, or move.*

~ Dov Davidoff

How are you sleeping?

As you've picked up this book, I could assume the answer is "not well". It's an important question to start with though.

When a baby is born, and visitors turn up en masse to meet the new arrival, one of the first questions people always seem to ask is if the little one is a good sleeper.

It may be out of concern for the parents, and to check that the baby isn't unknowingly and unintentionally depriving them of sleep. (Part of me thinks it's so they can tell you how *their* child sleeps much better than your child, or on the flip side, that they have it *way* worse than you. Either way social comparisons can be really unhelpful, especially to new parents.)

As an adult, asking how you're sleeping isn't something that comes up in general conversation. In the days before face masks and our movements restricted, if you bumped in to a group of friends on the High Street, the last (and definitely not the first) thing you might say is, "Did you sleep well last night?"

Although I do.

In my work as a counsellor, I ask about sleep because it's directly connected to how you're feeling right now, and is a doorway to what might be going on underneath. Your mood and your sleep are two sides of the same coin.

My professional journey of learning about sleep began right at the beginning of my therapeutic career, when I was fortunate enough to meet a qualified sleep specialist in the UK, who ran a professional sleep clinic near Cambridge, England. (His name was Martin and he later gave me an authorised tour of the facility, where the most fantastic equipment monitored sleep in all its forms. It was genuinely riveting.)

At the time, Martin was offering insights through workshops on the subject of sleep through a course he'd entitled "Faulty Winks". The training was for professionals who had an interest in the subject, and who wanted to help their clients understand the science behind what was getting in the way of proper shut-eye.

Around that time, I was becoming a qualified counsellor, spending three years learning a model of work referred to as "person centred" by the American psychologist Carl Rogers.

My professional training focused on the premise that if people felt they could share their fears and frustrations safely and non-judgementally in the counselling room – with what Rogers defined as Unconditional Positive Regard – purposeful, therapeutic work and recovery would take place.

At the time, I had also joined an agency that provided grief support and, from the outset, the majority of clients I worked with were bereaved by murder or suicide (in some cases both).

From the beginning of my therapeutic career I noticed two things about the work: 1) When the time was right for them, my clients wanted to find healthy and proactive ways to get what I refer to as their "sparkle" back. This would often include identifying ways to get a better night's sleep. And: 2) People wanted to talk to me about the dreams they were having.

Using my counselling training, and having investigated many dream theories like those of (but not limited to) Carl Jung – an early student of Sigmund Freud who ultimately challenged Freud's work – I began meaningful conversations of exploration with my clients at their request, about the dreams they would share with me.

Learning how to manage sleep, and unpacking their dreams or nightmares, helped my clients understand themselves in new ways, creating a pathway for recovery and healing. In many cases they have been able to consider the positive message their dreams contained, even when at first the content seemed confusing – even terrifying.

## The World Outside

My interest and passion for dream discovery started long before I qualified though.

I was born in the 70s, mum and dad divorced when I was tiny, and not long after the split we moved to Scotland for a while, then back to England a few years later.

We lived on a council estate. I played a game called "42-and-out" with my friends. I got the bus to school. At the weekend, I attended Sunday School, and in the evenings watched *Family Fortunes* from the ironing basket (true story). I read *Smash Hits* and played Rick Astley on repeat. It was the days of *Crossroads* and *Top of the Pops*. To the outside world, we were a normal family.

Behind closed doors it felt more like a scene from *Charmed*.

We had a black cat.

A statue of Aphrodite in the front room.

When I came home from school, my mum would be using a Ouija board or reading the Tarot. I fell asleep to the sound of her using the I Ching, an ancient Chinese divination tool. (I can still remember the "clink" of the coins even now.)

From an early age, I was encouraged to consider a world outside of what I could see, in fact my mum's mantra, "Everything that is, isn't, and everything that isn't, is" (translation: nothing is what it seems), came to her in a dream.

I was asked over breakfast what dreams I'd had the night before, my mum offering explanations which included definitions from dream analysts of her day like Nerys Dee. (I still have Dee's book *Your Dreams and What They Mean*.)

It was only when I went to school, and spoke about dreams in the playground, that I realised mine wasn't your average suburban household.

Recalling and recording my own dreams started as a hobby. I once dreamt I was pushing Vin Diesel in a shopping trolley, and then there was the time I watched the plot of a *Scooby Doo* movie unfold (I've not met anyone else yet who has dreamt in cartoon).

These are not the types of dream you'd commonly find in a dream dictionary, and this amongst other things was what particularly piqued my interest. Dream dictionaries are generic; people aren't.

It made perfect sense then, with all I was learning about dreams as I got older, that I dug deeper into sleep too. Martin's Faulty Winks training was the logical next step.

## When Sleepy Winks are Faulty

If you've ever managed a great night's sleep, you'll know that feeling of bliss when you wake up: how refreshed you feel, and how life just seems a bit, well... easier.

You make better decisions.

You're less grumpy.

Things don't feel so heavy.

But for many people, as soon as they turn out the lights, their bed becomes a magical place that reminds them of all the things they haven't done today.

If, as soon as your head hits the pillow, your mind takes you, as I call it, "down the plug hole", before too long you can find yourself sinking in to a low mood or state of anxiety. It's the place in your mind that you manage to avoid during the day (usually by keeping busy), but which your thoughts drag you into at night. It's dark down there, and the sheer weight of your thoughts can make it harder to climb back up.

On the surface of it, sleep can be a problem for all sorts of different reasons. If you're drinking lots of energy drinks or gallons of coffee every day, that's going to have an impact. I once met a lady who told me it was part of her job to make her boss's coffee every day. She decided to keep a work tracker to calculate how she was spending her time, because she didn't seem to be getting anything done. When she looked at it, she discovered she was making her boss a coffee every *nineteen* minutes.

Another person told me that they used to keep a *crate* of energy drinks in the boot of their car. This is how people feel they have to survive today.

I've mentioned already that top tips tend to focus on what you drink, and whether you own a lavender pillow spray.

But here's the thing: that might just be scratching the surface. The causes might also be:

- A stressful job.
- An elderly relative who's unwell.
- Family or financial worries.

And so much more.

Stress is regularly reported as the largest trigger for poor sleep, with women being more affected by life stress (52 per cent) than work stress (42 per cent).[9] Ditching the energy drinks won't necessarily help with all that's going on.

I will be unpacking this more, because I believe our inability to drift off is largely rooted somewhere else.

Where magazines and Internet searches try to blame poor sleep on lifestyle, I will argue the case that real sleep problems could go much deeper than that. Let's look at some myths around sleep first in case they help, before we dive in.

**Activity:** Start to think about what is really keeping you awake. You might want to look in the Sleep Cycle Repair Kit at the back, including Sleep Hygiene, to see if it's a daytime habit that's not helping. If, however, you think it might be something else, jot down in your journal just a few words to begin with. You don't need to dive deep just yet, but if it brings up difficult things then make sure you do this with support close by. Come back to this later if you're not sure yet.

# The Big Myths of Sleep

#1: *Everyone needs eight hours sleep.*
Reality: No, they don't.

The Internet is wonderful for so many reasons.

It makes access to information easier. We can get answers to questions when our mind goes blank and, if finances allow, order something for the kitchen at the touch of a button.

When I'm sat in front of the TV wondering what film I've seen that actor in before, or who sang a particular song, I no longer have to let it prod away at my mind for hours on end. I literally just type the question into my smartphone... and voila.

We can talk with friends and family, run businesses around the world, and order our weekly shop because of its capability; COVID-19 has made the Internet invaluable to those who have access to it.

The Coronavirus outbreak meant we had to swiftly change how we interact on a global scale, relying heavily on the Internet. Without it many of us wouldn't have been able to do our jobs, "see" our shielding loved ones, or find the answers to the office Zoom Pub Quiz.

However, one of the challenges of having knowledge so readily available on the web, is that information gets repeated as if it's fact. People accept it with certainty. Misinformation breeds. It then gets repeated over and over again without being challenged.

Big brands also endorse the idea that they have what you need to make you better. Some bed manufacturers, for example, advertise that you can speak to one of their "sleep gurus", who will offer you the same advice you could probably read in any magazine, but will sell you one of their duvets, pillows or mattresses as part of the deal.

It sounds cynical but insomnia is big business, not least of all because it's such a talking point.

There are currently more than 26.9 million posts using the hashtag #sleep on Instagram and if you use a search engine like Google, more than 2,890,000,000 results come up when you put in the same word.[10]

When Arianna Huffington was researching *The Sleep Revolution*, five thousand apps appeared when she searched sleep on the Apple App Store.[11] Companies, especially the pharmaceutical industry, are making big bucks. She explains:

*An entire industry has arisen to facilitate our attempts to get more sleep. A survey by Parade magazine of more than fifteen thousand people found that 23 per cent of respondents took sleeping pills once a week, and 14 per cent took them every night. The problem is global: in 2014, people around the world spent a staggering $58 billion on sleep aid products... for the drug industry that stands to profit from today's sleep crisis, business is good and the future looks bright.*

Because insomnia is good for the economy, it makes sense for large organisations to perpetuate some of the biggest myths.

One of those seems to be that you *must* get eight hours sleep *every* night. But it's just not that simple.

Yes, we *do* need to sleep. We know if we're not getting enough of it, it takes its toll. An article in *Psychology Today* identified that young people are more depressed than ever, not just because of what they see online but through sleep deprivation.[12]

But the myths around sleep are widespread, and in my view can do more harm than good. To highlight how far this goes, whenever I've travelled round the UK, I've asked thousands of people how much sleep they believe they *should* get according to what they've heard – they invariably answer "eight hours". (Some even say nine.)

The reality is, most of us aren't getting anywhere near that amount. According to one report,[13] a third of the population (33 per cent) now get by on five to six hours sleep, and 70 per cent of British people get less than seven.

But we worry about it. Believe it or not, thinking that you *need* eight hours sleep every night – especially in one solid block – could actually be one of the things that's keeping you awake. Research backs this up.

According to one survey, 79 per cent of people in the UK are lying awake at night worrying how long they've been awake, and whether they're going to get the recommended amount.[14]

We've become so programmed with the idea that we *have* to have the right amount, that people now calculate what time they go to bed, based on what time they need to set their alarm and subtracting eight. If a person needs to get up at 6am, they'll work back eight hours and figure they've got to be in bed by 10pm.

But your body doesn't work like that (more on that in Myth #2). And this myth is really having an impact.

When people wake up in the middle of the night, the first thing they usually do is check their phone – why? Because they want to see what time it is, and work out how many hours they can get in before they have to get up.

When people work out their bedtime based on the formula:

mandatory wake time minus eight

they then wonder why they can't get to sleep. And when they don't sleep well, they think they've done something wrong, or that they're just rubbish at it. As human beings we don't like to fail at anything.

When something goes wrong, we instinctively adopt what I know as the At Fault Position. We instantly take the blame, assuming it must be something we're doing – or not doing right. Someone crashes into you in the supermarket with their shopping cart or trolley – what's the first thing you say? "Sorry." That's the At Fault Position in action.

When I've asked people why they think their sleeping tablets, anti-anxiety pills or antidepressants aren't working, they tell me there must be something wrong with themselves; that's the only logical conclusion they can reach. They don't assume the information, treatment option or advice they've been given is possibly incorrect, not personally relevant, or even misleading. So they don't challenge it, and persevere with something that's just not working.

A former president of the Sleep Research Society, Jerome Siegel discovered in a study of pre-industrial societies the amount of sleep people need varies from person to person, with some needing only 5.7 hours a night.[15] The amount of sleep we need varies dependent on our age and on what's happening in our lives.

When we're poorly we need more sleep; it is often described as the best medicine.[16] Children need more sleep than adults because of their ongoing development; newborns might easily sleep 16 hours+ a day. Teenagers also need more sleep, especially when they're studying.

According to the Sleep Foundation, teens can easily average 10 hours sleep a night; the benefits include sharper thinking, spurring creativity and recognising the most important information to consolidate learning.

*Whether it's studying for a test, learning an instrument, or acquiring job skills, sleep is essential for teens.*[17]

(This means, to bust another myth, teenagers are not lazy if they're laying in more often – they really do need their sleep.)

A person in later life might be quite satisfied on six hours decent kip. The late Margaret Thatcher, the first female British

Prime Minister, reportedly used to say she could get by on just three or four (she also apparently said "sleep is for wimps").

People do wake up on less than eight hours sleep and be full of the joys of spring. If this is you, and you don't need any stimulants (like coffee, or energy drinks) to keep you firing on all cylinders, and you're not suffering from any ill effects of less sleep (like always getting ill, can't concentrate, often forgetful, feeling low) then hopefully this chapter encourages you that it's okay you're not getting a full eight hours in.

If you feel fine both physically and mentally, you sleep enough to get some decent dreaming in, and it's just the *thought* of not getting eight hours that's stressing you out, then ditch the myth.

But if you're one of millions of people who feel shattered whether you get eight hours or 10, or if it feels unhealthy to be getting less than that, read on.

In summary then:

The eight-hour narrative appears to have created problems of its own.

The majority of us aren't achieving eight hours sleep. We worry about it, so we can't doze off. It becomes a vicious cycle.

If you're laying in bed and your mind goes in to a tailspin with worries about –

- what you'll feel like in the morning if you don't sleep
- how you're not going to be able to concentrate the next day
- missing the alarm
- being late for work
- having an accident because you're so tired

– this may all be because of the eight-hour myth.

Sleep is more about quality than quantity, and considering what's happening in your life at the time.

Remember, if sleep deprivation is really taking its toll, if you are struggling with sleep right now, and feel you need to ask for medical help, please do that. If you're not sleeping at all, or getting less than six hours a night on a regular basis and it's making you unwell, reach out to your doctor to see if they can help you work out what's going on.

For our next myth, we're going to look at when you *should* be going to bed.

*Nod to Broken Sleep Technology: A study published in the* Journal of Clinical Sleep Medicine *describes a new sleep disorder arising from the pursuit of a perfect night's sleep.*[18]

*"Orthosomnia" ("ortho" meaning straight or correct, "somnia" meaning sleep) affects people who obsess over the results of their sleep and fitness tracker, which ironically can affect their rest.*

*The researchers explained: "Relying solely on the data on their trackers, people are convincing themselves that they suffer from a sleep disorder, even when they may not. The subsequent outcome is people who are becoming obsessed with getting a 'perfect' night's sleep."*

*The best way to tell how well you slept, is how refreshed you feel the next day.*

**Activity:** If it's helpful you could use your journal for the next week to begin noting how refreshed you feel when you wake up, on a scale of 1-10 (1 is not at all, 10 is amazing). There's an activity at the back on how to keep a more detailed sleep diary.

## Time

*Time is priceless yet it costs us nothing.*
*You can do anything you want with it, but you can't own it.*
*You can spend it but you can't keep it.*
*And once you've lost it, there's no getting it back.*
*It's just gone.*
~ taken from the TV Show, *Medium*

# The Big Myths of Sleep

#2: *Bedtime is a specific time.*
Reality: No, it's not.

As a society, we love to talk about time; more specifically, that there never seems to be enough of it, and how we are always rushing around.

Ask anyone you meet the question, "How are you?" and invariably, when they don't reply with the social mandate, "I'm fine," they'll say something like, "I'm so busy."

As companies adapt their hierarchies from being less manager-led to more task driven, social status – which for a long time has been in part defined by your job title – is now determined by how busy you are. How packed your calendar is, equates to how important you must be.

In the 21st Century, we carry busy-ness as a badge of honour with an unwritten rule book that says, whatever you do, you mustn't waste time. This is just one reason why sleep could be posing a problem for so many.

Although evidence suggests FOMO (the Fear Of Missing Out) has been around for centuries,[19] it is now being recognised as an anxiety caused by the societal pressure to keep up with everyone else, in case they're having more fun. Our need to be involved in the world around us is made possible – and at the same time worse – by access to information and people 24/7.

Because sleep has the potential to swallow up hours of our time, the idea of wasting precious amounts of it overnight feels almost socially taboo.

It's one reason I think people apologise if they feel they have to go to bed early, as if they're doing something wrong. I've genuinely taught in classrooms where I've seen people feel ashamed or embarrassed to admit in front of others that they're usually crashed out in bed by 9pm.

The arrival of the Industrial Age may well have changed the way we think about sleep today. The American inventor and businessman, Thomas Edison, was quoted as saying, "Sleep is a criminal waste of time, inherited from our cave days."

Although it has profound benefits, like improving memory and concentration, maintaining a healthy weight, and keeping our immune system strong,[20] unless you enjoy sleep, it can feel like an absolute chore.

I've heard people say they believe they'd get *so* much more done, if they didn't have to sleep. I once met a lady who told me that going to sleep and going to the toilet were two of the biggest wastes of her time every day. She said if she could manifest a way that she didn't have to do either (basically so she could stay at her desk and work), she would do it.

These examples highlight the strength of our relationship with time and how, as human beings, we are obsessed with it – even if it's to the detriment of our health. And it's something quite unique to the human race.

In his gorgeous story *The Time Keeper*, Mitch Albom writes:

*Try to imagine a life without timekeeping. You probably can't. You know the month, the year, the day of the week. There is a clock on your wall or the dashboard of your car. You have a schedule, a calendar, a time for dinner or a movie. Yet all around you, timekeeping is ignored. Birds are not late. A dog does not check its watch. Deer do not fret over passing birthdays. Man alone measures time. Man alone chimes the hour. And, because of this, man alone suffers a paralysing fear that no other creature endures. A fear of time running out.*

Time dominates our lives and the fear of wasting it seeps into our consciousness from a young age. If you were ever caught sitting doing nothing as a child, you might have been called lazy, the implication being that you should be doing something *more* with your time, than having what may actually be a well-deserved rest.

As science continues to explore the purpose of sleep, studies have also been conducted to see whether or not we can get by with no sleep at all.

When the military have tried to teach even the "toughest people on the planet" to go without sleep, after three days Navy Seals reported hallucinating.[21] Doctors, nurses and other front-line personnel will also know the longer-term impact of complete sleep deprivation.

Even those who don't work shifts, or resist sleep for whatever reason, can still fear the consequences of not getting enough of it and, as we saw in Myth #1, worry starts to infiltrate our thinking, in case it impacts our eight hours.

I mentioned earlier, when we wake up in the night we usually look at the clock to see how much time is left before we have to get up. Generally speaking, we only do this because we're worried that time will affect us in some way. If it's still dark, we might fret about wasting time awake because we're in bed and we "should" be asleep. If it's almost dawn, we might write off getting any more sleep at all.

It's one of the reasons when people wake up and it's dark outside, they get up – even if it's the middle of the night – because they figure they might as well do something useful.

A lady once told me she'd get through an entire pile of ironing in the middle of the night, and another would wash her windows from top to bottom. (I'll come on to explain in *The 4am Mystery*, why getting up in the night can also be part of the problem, unless you really need to do it.)

The idea of being up in the night when we think we should be asleep causes us to do things which, ironically, keep us awake. Our brain is stimulated, tricked even, into thinking it's time to get up, even though it can feel like absolute torture when you're shattered, especially the next day. No one I've met has ever told me they woke up in the middle of the night and said with genuine excitement, as they turn to look at the clock, "Yippee, it's 2am!"

Unless you're getting up in the middle of the night to catch a flight (which, due to COVID, will be up in the air if you'll pardon the pun), no one *really* wants to know what time it is. But it doesn't stop us looking.

Whilst the continued improvement of modern technology has developed immense possibilities, most noticeably since the Coronavirus outbreak, it has also meant a loss of our most basic wisdom, such as knowing when to go to bed.

When I ask people that very question – "When do you go to bed?" – they always answer with a specific time. They never say, "When I'm sleepy."

This is a key point.

Our body isn't really wired to work on Industrial Time, and yet many of us are using the clock to determine how we operate it. We set a time for lunch, even if we're not hungry. We make a brew for "elevenses" (just because). And we try to convince our body when it's time for bed.

As I introduced in the last myth, we use the calculation of:

wake time minus eight = bedtime.

However, this is not a reliable method of determining when we *need* to go to sleep. Essentially, we try to make the needs of our body fit around our working day, but we don't seem to have evolved quickly enough that we can thrive that way. As a result, our bodies and natural rhythms are out of sync with the world around us.

Before the onset of the Industrial Revolution, our days revolved around cycles, whether it was the sun, the moon or seasons. The tolling of bells were only used to call parishioners to church services or warn of calamities or celebrations.[22] In colder months we'd hibernate; with warmer weather, we'd sow and harvest.

The replacement of hand tools with power-driven machinery meant success wasn't measured by how well fed and settled we were. It became more aligned with how much we had and how much we could get done. Sleep became unfavourable. Inconvenient. A problem.

When analogue clocks became more reliable in the 1800s and sundials became obsolete,[23] we tried to slot our lives neatly and conveniently in to three portions of eight: one for work, one for play, and one for rest. (The eight-hour working day was always meant to be a good thing, to prevent abuse of power within labour markets, especially for children.[24] It's since become another rule book to live by.)

As technology advances, and we are now available to our employers around the clock, we have less time for leisure and rest, and we spend more time on work. According to one YouGov poll, six out of 10 people check their emails on holiday.[25]

Instead of resting in the winter months where we would enjoy the fruits of our labours, we now wrench ourselves out of bed on a cold December morning to get more done.

And we're so tired.

Our valiant efforts to tell our bodies when to sleep (only because that's when it's convenient), aren't working.

Just as King Canute couldn't stop the tide, you can't control something cyclic when nature's got the wheel.

Although your brain is not really like a computer,[26] evolutionarily speaking if it did have an operating system we might say it hasn't had an upgrade in quite some time. Whilst with good intentions, we may tell ourselves that 10pm is the bedtime we're aiming for, it won't work if your body – or your mind – is not ready to rest.

Essentially, the process of sleep is governed by different factors that need to align. These include onset of darkness and whether the environment you're in lends itself to nodding off. (Siegel for example, who I mentioned earlier, said temperature matters – the cooler the better – which would explain why we struggle to sleep during a heatwave. I'll talk about bedroom environment later.)

As the day goes on and the evening rolls in, your brain monitors the environment and the production of melatonin begins, contributing towards feelings of sleepiness. If it's safe, calm, cool and quiet, and night-time's arriving, your body's probably going to start gearing up for sleep.

However, unnatural light – like the blue light that comes from your TV or your mobile phone – mimics the sun and can suppress melatonin because it still registers as light in the brain. Even "Blue Light Filters", designed so you can keep using your phone in to the night, don't always work: probably because light is light. Your brain registers it's not dark, thinks you're looking at the sun, and decides the time for sleep has ended.

This is why you don't always feel sleepy even though you're tired; being sleepy and tiredness are not the same thing. You'll know this yourself if you've ever fallen in to bed, absolutely worn out after an exhausting day, and then be surprised – if not frustrated – when sleep doesn't arrive.

And there's more.

Sleep is like a bus: if you miss it, you might have to wait for the next one.

## The Bus Route

I appreciate it might sound a bit random, but I created this analogy to help explain one of the reasons I believe people can't sleep at the specific time they want or try to, even though they're *really* tired. (Remember, tiredness and sleepiness are not the same.)

Buses have timetables and so does your body: the 24-hour rhythm we know as circadian, and the shorter cycles (like a sleep cycle) known as ultradian. Knowing when sleep (the bus) is on its way can help you organise your bedtime, and create a plan in case you miss it.

Contrary to what we might have been led to believe, when we go to bed isn't so much a specific *hour*. If we had to narrow it down, the "best" time is quoted as somewhere between 9pm and 11pm. (This doesn't help people who, for example, work shifts though. I'll come on to this too.)

Here's what we do know:

The sleep cycle in adults lasts about 90 to 120 minutes. (It's shorter in young children, between 45-60 minutes depending on their age.) This means, in this analogy, your bus comes round every couple of hours, but like most timetables, there's some give and take.

Like catching a bus, there's a rough window of opportunity to catch your z's, only in this case it's not what it says on the clock. It's when you might feel your eyes drooping or your head nodding. This can be a sign of what's called Sleep Pressure.

If your body is registering sleepiness at 9pm but you decide to stay up an hour because *Game of Thrones* is on, when you go to bed 60 minutes later you might find you're wide awake. How is this possible, when just an hour before you were sleepy?

It might be because the blue light from the telly registered as daylight and suppressed melatonin, or the action from the TV show stimulated you in to thinking what was happening on screen could happen to you (a style of unconscious mirroring).

It might also be that, like a bus, there is a window of opportunity to catch sleep from when you start to feel sleepy – clients usually report the window is open for around 20-35(ish) minutes. What this means is, we have our own personal bedtime unique to each of us – and it's less to do with time, more with how you feel. But, because people tend to push through their sleepiness, when they do eventually go to bed (in this example an hour later when *Game of Thrones* has finished) they can't sleep. So the key message here is go to bed when you start to feel sleepy, rather than putting it off for too long, as you might be awake a while longer if you don't.

When I've talked about this with the hundreds of people I've worked with and used my analogy of buses, they've said it made perfect sense. When they went to bed as soon as they started to feel sleepy, they slept much better (they caught "the bus"). If they pushed through it, and went to bed an hour later, they'd find they couldn't sleep (they'd missed it). When they did feel sleepy again, it was about an hour and a half to two hours from when they first felt like they could have gone to bed. Incidentally, this may also be one reason why if you try to put a child to bed too early, i.e. when they're not sleepy, they'll be up for a while yet. Kids not only have a sleep cycle, they may have a window of opportunity too.

Just to make these points, I describe one scenario, from Elena, like many I've heard:

*A normal evening for me is that I usually feel sleepy around 9.30pm-ish – my eyes feel heavy, but I usually push through it as I still have things to do. I do all my jobs in the evening, so before I go up to bed I feed the cat, do the washing up and then head upstairs. Then I brush my teeth, take off my make-up, put my pyjamas on and so on. I'm not doing anything too taxing, so I always think I'll just drop off because I felt so sleepy just half an hour before, but when I try to sleep I can't. Now I know why!*

Elena noticed after we spoke that she started to feel sleepy again around 11pm (90-120 minutes – the length of a sleep cycle – after she first felt like she could have gone to bed). Prior to this Elena would toss and turn in bed from 10pm, getting more and more wound up that she couldn't sleep. Now, she says, she either goes to bed when she feels sleepy at 9.30pm, or later when she feels she'll nod off.

Many people like Elena, before they heard this analogy, would get stressed worrying about Myth #1 – that they're not going to get their eight hours – or frustrated when they don't drift off even though they felt sleepy only half an hour before.

The more stressed we become (and the more we shout at our brain or body for not playing ball), the less likely we are to sleep. The activation of our "fight or flight" response is never going to authorise shut-eye when you're feeling troubled or distressed. Like many others, Elena would find herself so stressed that she wasn't sleeping, ironically it would keep her awake.

Here's another example from Lola, after we talked about this:

*I used to fall asleep in front of the TV, my eyelids go and that's it. I'll wake up about two hours later, with the telly still blaring. So I get up, close the curtains, do some bits and bobs around the house, then eventually go to bed about half an hour or so later. But then I can't sleep. It made no sense to me, until now.*

After we spoke, Lola took the decision not to fall asleep in front of the TV anymore, and instead head to bed when her eyelids started to droop. As a result, she says her sleep improved dramatically.

Note also that Lola was waking up in front of the telly a couple of hours after she had felt sleepy – the rough length of a sleep cycle. However, because before Lola and I had spoken, she had previously gone straight in to "busy-ness" as soon as she woke up, she had missed the bus. (If you're really interested, you can track the length of your sleep cycle on paper by noting your sleep/wake times – i.e. without using an app. Just know these can vary though.)

Any sort of activity that stimulates your thought processes – not just stress or busy-ness – can trick the brain into thinking you need to stay awake, when it's actually time for bed.

One couple once told me that, no matter what they did, they couldn't get to sleep at night, even though they'd gone to bed tired. I asked them, without going in to too much detail, what they did just before they tried to sleep and they told me they would do a puzzle, like a word search or a crossword. They'd get their puzzle books out and see who would win first and then, once finished, find they couldn't sleep.

As innocent and meaningful as it was to share a moment of harmless fun together, it was stimulating their brains. A sense of competition – where there is the potential for a winner and a loser – can be enough to get their competitive juices flowing, and thereby potentially keep them both awake. Your body doesn't just need darkness to sleep, it needs a calm, uncompetitive environment too.

It also needs to respond to the calls of nature, even in the dark. Here's another example of how the bus fits in.

A couple of years ago, when I was teaching a course on dreams, a guest I'll call Granger told me his situation.

Granger explained that for years, he had been waking up in the night because he needed the loo, even if he'd cut down on drinks before bedtime.

He described how he'd start to stir, realise he needed to go but because he was warm and cozy in bed, he'd try to prioritise sleep and comfort over the need to empty his bladder.

Eventually, he would have to get up because Mother Nature called and She doesn't wait for anyone. So after half an hour of putting it off, he'd go to the loo only then to find, when he got back in to bed, he couldn't sleep for at least another hour or so.

I explained my bus analogy to him and the idea of a window of opportunity, which seems to apply in the same way if you need to go back to sleep, as it does if you're having trouble dropping off in the first place.

In Granger's case, him trying to put off answering the

call of nature meant that he was pushing into – and out of – that window of sleepiness. Because he'd taken so much time deciding whether to get up or not, which actually stressed him out, inevitably he only found that when he did get back in to bed, he'd missed the bus.

I simply suggested that Granger try getting up as soon as he realised he needed the loo, then getting back in to bed. He came back the following week and the exact word he used was that it had been "revolutionary".

When Granger woke up needing a pee, he was still sleepy. By getting up straight away, having a tiddle, no drama, and then getting back in to bed, he stayed within the window of opportunity, and didn't stress himself out. Instead of delaying getting up, he now simply wakes up, heads to the loo, gets back in to bed and falls straight back to sleep. Sleeping when you're sleepy is key, not what the clock says.

Now, you might say to me (as some people have), "Well this is all very well, Delphi, but if it's a case of going to bed when I'm sleepy, I'll be heading for bed at 7pm!" And I hear you.

Early evening sleepiness might mean that lack of sleep is catching up with you, especially if you've noticed a tendency or real desire to drift off doing your day job. According to the Big Sleep Report,[27] 12 per cent of people also admitted falling asleep during a workplace meeting.

The good news is that when you follow a more natural approach to bedtime and understand some of these myths, you might find the time you go to bed evens out to something you feel is more socially acceptable.

If the bus analogy applies, with your sleep cycle lasting an hour and a half to two hours, keep in mind that if you do feel sleepy at 7pm but don't go to bed, you will feel sleepy again as Sleep Pressure builds, as long as you don't keep "pushing through" and the rest of your environment lends itself to rest.

The bus analogy could also work for people who do night shifts as long as the conditions are right for sleep. If you have to sleep during the day make sure your bedroom is calm, quiet and dark enough so that your body registers that it's time for bed.

Some employers will keep the lights low for people in warehouses so as not to overstimulate the brain (and under stimulate melatonin production), and may even supply special glasses so that when you leave work you're not walking out in to the glaring sun; ask your boss if they can help. Power naps can also be valuable if you work shifts, more on this later too.

The key message is go to bed when you're sleepy when you can, and try not to place the emphasis on what time it is. The majority of people I meet are using the clock and the eight-hour myth to dictate their sleep habits, calculating when they should go to bed, and how many hours sleep they can achieve before the alarm goes off; these alone as we've seen can create problems.

In all the years I've been talking about this, I've only ever met two people who said the theory behind my bus analogy – the idea of going to bed when you are sleepy – didn't work for them. They said they noticed that as soon as they felt sleepy they felt they *had* to go to bed but had too much to do, and ironically that caused them stress; your brain won't let you sleep when you're putting pressure on yourself to do so. So it wasn't the "bus timetable" that stressed them out so much, but more likely their thoughts about it.

If busting this myth or talking about buses doesn't work for you don't worry, take a look at what's next.

Another myth is the belief that it's wrong to wake up in the night.

**Activity:** When you next have some time off, ideally over a seven-day period, see if you notice when you feel naturally sleepy and when you wake up without an alarm. This could help you work out your natural bed/wake time. (You may have noticed this already since the Coronavirus outbreak.)

*Nod to Mental Health: There is a direct relationship between sleep and poor mental health, which can become a vicious cycle. The more you don't sleep, the more stressed you may feel; the more stressed you feel, the less likely you'll sleep.*

*According to the Mental Health Foundation, the average person gets asked how are you 14 times a week. When someone says, "I'm fine," they only mean it 19 per cent of the time. That means when someone tells you they're okay, 81 per cent of the time, they don't feel able to talk about how they feel.*

*When you ask someone how they are in future, if you really want to know, ask again with, "How are you really?"[28] Or even follow up with, "How are you sleeping?"*

# The Big Myths of Sleep

#3: *Waking up at night is unnatural.*
Reality: No, it's not.

How many times have you woken up in the middle of the night, for no apparent reason, your heart sank and you thought "not this again!"? If you do, you're not alone.

I described earlier the At Fault Position, where we automatically assume we are to blame when something goes wrong. This means, when people wake up at night, they draw the conclusion it must be something they've done. People have come to believe that waking up at night is bad, when in fact it's a healthy and natural thing.

In Granger's case it was the physical need to go to the loo that woke him up; if he hadn't stirred and realised what he needed, we can probably all guess what might have happened. We wake up in the night for all sorts of reasons, not just the call of nature, including physical and emotional pain. But people are often frustrated or panic if they wake up even once, because they think it's not right.

As well as Myth #1, believing that we *need* to get eight hours sleep *every* night, society also seems to think that when we do sleep it should be in a solid, unbreakable chunk. The reality is, most people don't always sleep straight through and there's nothing unnatural about it.

I am going to talk about buses *briefly* again.

I mentioned in Myth #2 that to me, sleep is like a bus, the cycle like a route. We know that during each cycle throughout the night the bus travels a journey (in the form of stages), and you'll start to feel sleepy especially as the night draws in.

We know we sleep in stages thanks to the work of Dement and others and, for the purposes of this book, I'm going to describe them as light sleep, deep sleep and Rapid Eye Movement (REM) sleep – each one moves round to the next. After light sleep comes deep sleep, then REM and so it repeats, basically in that order. (There's more on this in the Kit later too.)

If you're someone that has no trouble falling asleep, but notices you wake up several times in the night, you might notice that you're waking up every hour and a half (or thereabouts) but manage to doze off again. Some people know that they wake up, some people don't. It's often the people who know they wake up in the night that struggle, mainly because they think it's *wrong*.

In fact, science would suggest it's perfectly natural to wake up at night, even essential to our survival.

As we move out of dreaming sleep and back round in to lighter sleep, it's quite normal if there is a brief awareness of awakening. It's one of the reasons why people wake up with a dream or nightmare, but can then roll over and go back to sleep.

In science-y speak it's called Sleep Arousal, and not the morning glory kind. It's just the term to describe the normal natural waking as we transition through the phases of sleep.

To emphasise this point, it's not even the waking up that's the problem – it's what we do next.

It's when we wake up and beat ourselves up, tell ourselves off, blame our body, shout at the cat, and get caught in a spiral of thinking about how life *should* be (see *Going Down the Plughole*) that stops us going back to sleep.

If you woke up last night, you might be one of the people who has an awareness of awakening as you come to the end of a natural sleep cycle before the next one begins. There's nothing wrong with that. Instead of cursing into the darkness, you can actually just acknowledge you're awake, that it's just how it is, and drift back off in to the land of nod. If that doesn't convince you, read on.

The reason we wake up in the night might also be a survival

mechanism, especially if there's a lot going on for you right now, where your brain is just "checking in" that everything's as it should be. When we're hyper vigilant, stressed or upset, it makes perfect sense that there's a part of our brain on sentry duty, like a guard at Buckingham Palace, just to check you're safe and sound.

Rather than this process of waking being unnatural then or – as some might see it – the enemy, your brain is engaged in a natural internal safety check that's looking for a green light that everything's okay.

It's not a new thing, it's been around long before the arrival of smartphones, Netflix and Amazon Prime, although their invention won't have helped if the first thing we do when we wake up is check to see what time it is (see Myth #2).

The only real exception to this, might be if you're someone who is regularly waking up, and your sleep is so disrupted, in which case it's time to ask the doctor for help. Even then, there are lots of reasons this might be, and some of them easily fixed.

We can develop a "habit" of not sleeping well, and like most habits they can be broken, or at least replaced with healthier ones. If your sleep has become so disrupted, it might be your body is out of sync with natural rhythms, and your brain just doesn't know what's normal anymore.

Your doctor might arrange for you to visit a laboratory, to examine your actual sleep activity. This sounds way more scientific than it actually is, and having seen one I can say they're not a place to be scared about; they are really cool places. (Think *Big Bang Theory*, rather than Frankenstein's Den.)

Under these controlled conditions, people often discover that they were actually asleep more than they thought, in fact what they're remembering are the brief moments they were awake – the normal "arousals" I mentioned earlier, that just felt longer than they were. (The passing of time can appear skewed in the middle of the night.)

There are various, rare sleep disorders that can affect your natural sleep patterns which again can be managed well, some even without any long-term medication. I'm not going to go in to them in this book because, like I say, this is not that sort of a book. But do chat to your doctor and see how they can help. And if your doctor's not sympathetic, organisations like Healthwatch (in the UK) may be able to advocate on your behalf.

Middle of the night waking might also have something to do with what I talked about earlier, around time. When we try to put the round peg of Agricultural Time (the days before clocks and factories), which we lived by for millennia, in to the square peg of industrialism, our Stone Age brains try to keep up with a relatively new idea that we need a solid block of eight hours when it just wasn't designed like that. So we get stressed about it, when in fact as I alluded to a moment ago, our night-time waking might in fact be a basic, essential survival mechanism.

In the days when we lived in caves, some believe we would wake up several times during the night, just to check no one had stolen our food or, worse, our children. In a study of the Hadza tribe in Tanzania, by David Samson at Duke University,[29] at least one member of the group stays "aware" at night to protect the tribe, described as Nighttime Vigilance. Samson explains this "sentinel" behaviour could also be why teenagers tend to be awake later in to the night, whereas older people wake up earlier the next day.

It's generally agreed that sleeping all night in those days wasn't safe, and for many people today this survival instinct feels just as relevant as it was thousands of years ago.

Although we may think waking up in the dark is the nightmare, it could well be the brain just doing its job. If your thoughts reflect where your head is at during the day, it makes sense your survival instincts kick in at night if you're stressed, anxious or feeling depressed.

Although it might be more convenient to achieve solid chunks of sleep, so that it fits in with our busy 24/7 lives, the governing part of our brain that looks after our survival isn't quite there yet.

So if you're someone who thinks you're failing at life because you're waking up in the middle of the night, I want to reassure you first and foremost, that it's more likely you're functioning as a human being, and your brain is looking out for you.

Even if life feels completely dysfunctional right now, it might help to know that waking up at night might just be your brain's way of protecting you.

Because everyone is different, some people sleep through the night without noticing they wake up, others do. In Siegel's study, I mentioned in Myth #1, he found some pre-industrial societies did sleep through the night, although he acknowledged more research needed to be done. Whereas in Samson's research described above, at least one person in the household could potentially find themselves awake each night.

Your body is built to withstand certain periods of poor sleep, without any long-term lasting effects. New parents have bouts of interrupted sleep for weeks on end, which is normal and usually manageable over time. If you've had a bereavement, you'll know that for the first couple of weeks *at least*, sleep isn't something that comes naturally.

So, waking up in the night is normal, and may even be a "sentinel reflex" to make sure your household is safe. If you do wake in the night, it's what you think about it that matters, and what you do next.

**Activity:** Mindfulness and Meditation has been proven particularly useful for people who wake up in the night. There are meditation activities to try later on in the book.

*Nod to Research: According to Claudia Aguirre's TED Talk,*[30] *in*

*1965 17-year-old Randy Gardner stayed awake for 264 hours – 11 days – to see how he'd cope without sleep. On the second day his eyes stopped focusing, and by day three he was described as moody and uncoordinated. By the end of the experiment he was paranoid and "hallucinating". He recovered without any long-term effects. (Please don't try this at home).*

# The 4am Mystery

*Four in the morning, crapped out, yawning...*
~ Paul Simon, *Still Crazy After All These Years* (Song)

The 4am mystery. That's an actual thing by the way.

At least, it's a phenomenon described by the poet Rives, who through his 2007 TED Talk suggested "something more" could be linked to 4am,[31] and why we're awake.

Whilst his talk may be received by some as more poetic philosophy than evidence of an actual reason we're awake, Rives impressively catalogues, in a light-hearted way, coincidences over nearly a century which mention four-in-the-morning as the time when something meaningful is going on.

Where Rives says he finds 4am the most placid and uneventful hour of the day, in the video he highlights how it gets a lot of bad press across the media. He says:

*It's become... some sort of shorthand that you are awake at the worst possible hour; a time for inconveniences, mishaps and yearnings.*

If you're someone who is regularly finding yourself awake, sometimes for what feels like no reason, you'll understand what Rives is getting at. Being awake in the middle of the night is at best annoying, and at worst, a time when emotions run high.

When it's hard to switch off your mind, or turn down the noise in your head (especially when it's extremely loud and seems unending), then it makes sense that people feel desperate about being awake. This is especially the case if, until now, you'd believed you *should* be getting eight hours every night or had lived by any of the other myths I've described in the previous pages.

Whether it's experiencing the heartache of loss, or battling periods of depression for years, the middle of the night can be a time when we feel distraught, bereft and hopeless; on a personal level, I myself can relate to this and I'll share my own experience of it later.

It's one of the reasons why, in my work as a counsellor, as well as taking obvious steps to make sure someone is safe, I advise people *never* to make an important decision in the middle of the night, especially when you feel like you can't take much more. The Samaritans are available to call on 116 123 – including the middle of the night – for exactly this reason.

I want to reassure you that instead of 4am (or any other time in the middle of the night) being the worst possible hour, there is hope.

## What Keeps Us Awake

I've talked about why we wake up in the night, but what is it that keeps us there? Over the years, I have heard and researched many theories about why that is, and I've mentioned some already.

It could be something practical, like it was with Granger needing the loo. It could be you ate too much/too little or too late the night before; hunger can wake us up, just like indigestion can. (In one episode of *The Simpsons*, Homer makes reference to being awake at 4am on Christmas Day when his stomach's rumbling.) It might be our natural instinct of Nighttime Vigilance to check our loved ones are safe.

It might be an external click, buzz, whirr or hum from a clock, tap, street lamp or pylon, or even a health consideration like tinnitus. One lady who attended one of my mindfulness workshops said she suffered with this, and noticed it intensely at night. After attending a few sessions of the course, and learning how paying attention to sound through mindfulness can actually be quite relaxing, she said it didn't seem to bother her so much.

You might wake up because you thought you heard someone call your name, which I've included in a later section. Some might believe being woken up at night is a sign of spiritual awakening.[32]

Physical pain, hormones, blood sugars and temperature dropping can all be reasons that we rise in to consciousness in the dark hours. In her book *The Women's Guide to Overcoming Insomnia*, Shelby Harris writes:

> *Body temperature will continue to drop very slightly throughout the night-time hours as melatonin is released. The temperature will be at its lowest at around 3 or 4am, at which time melatonin is then essentially shutting off in the brain, helping the body become more alert as morning comes.*

If it's a dream or nightmare that's woken you up, it could be that something you're unable to focus on during the day is playing out in your sleep at night; dreaming is often described as night-time therapy; more on this later.

Watching a scary film before bed might give you a nightmare, and if it's bad enough, it might even make you afraid to sleep, or perhaps of the dark itself (the next chapter explains).

Some experts say if you were anxious at the time you watched a film, this can display itself in a bad dream. Watching a horror movie and then having a nightmare about it could also be your mind's way of relaying emotions you felt unable to express during the film.[33]

You might not know what it was that woke you up, and *that's* what becomes the focus of your attention. I mentioned in Myth #3 it's natural to wake up in the middle of the night; you may come in to wakefulness as you transition from dreaming sleep in to light sleep; if you can roll over and nod back off, there's no problem. However, if you start *thinking* about why you're awake it becomes one.

More than two decades ago, I woke up in the middle of the night for no obvious reason, and ended up walking round the house to see if I could find what it was that woke me up. Nothing was obviously wrong, but of course when I got back into bed, I couldn't sleep as my brain was now in Alert Mode; as I mentioned earlier, a stressed brain won't authorise sleep.

It could be you're struggling with loss, which isn't always in the shape of death, which I cover more in the chapter entitled *Under Grief*. When people have had a bereavement, they tell me how, when they wake up, just for a split second it feels like their loss isn't "real" – they have forgotten for a moment that their loved one is no longer here, and then it hits them. Understandably, moments like this would keep most people awake.

It might be something you can't really describe, like an ineffable sensation that you can't put words around. This is how some people describe anxiety, a noise in their head that often has no obvious storyline. For some, it's feelings of falling short, not measuring up or not being good enough in some way.

In her book *Tired But Wired*, Dr Nerina Ramlakhan says:

*We go into our shallowest stages of sleep around this time so if conditions aren't perfect for sleep we are more likely to wake. You are also more likely to wake in the early hours if you suffer from depression or anxiety.*

If any of these ring a bell with you, the Sleep Cycle Repair Kit might help but of course have a chat with your doctor if you feel a check-up might help.

One thing we know for sure is that emotions feel stronger, more powerful, more devastating at 4am. The whole world can feel darker.

The good news is, whilst we might have previously considered only one answer in the middle of the night, there may be many others to consider helpfully, which usually become apparent – or at least feel a little brighter – just as the sun rises.

So it's okay if you find yourself awake, and to acknowledge thoughts that might have led you there. Instead of becoming tangled in your thinking, you can learn how to become the observer of your thoughts rather than the participant, and this is where many find mindfulness can help.

You might choose to make a note of the epiphanies, and extraordinary moments of clarity you feel you're having at night, but *don't* ever feel you have to act on them, unless it's an emergency and you need to ring 999.

If you do find yourself awake in the middle of the night and life seems too difficult, you could also create a crisis or well-being plan before you go to bed, that will keep you safe until morning. This would include reaching out to people who can help (there's an example template at the end of the next chapter).

You *can* get through the darkness.

Day always follows night, and things usually feel better in the light of day.

I recognise that if you've been struggling to sleep for a long time, or been woken up by horrific nightmares that leave you crying or your heart pounding, you might be struggling with this logic; I hear you. But stay and work through it, with help if you need. Even though Rives approaches this with humour, he may well be on to something. The time we spend awake in the middle of the night could provide us with insights that could help build a better future; the dark may even become our friend and helper.

As well as describing 4am as the "worst possible hour", he also speaks of poets, writers and musicians who have referred to 4am as a key moment for reflection and introspection. Whilst night-time might feel like the enemy at the moment, Rives' insights suggest it brings with it a source of wisdom.

You don't have to be the writers and musicians he talks about, who get up in the middle of the night to write their masterpieces – although if it helps to get your words on to paper, try it. You certainly don't have to use the time you should be sleeping to get *more* jobs done, like the lady I mentioned earlier who would get up and do all her ironing. But you can make the darkness work for you.

Night-time is intended for rest, and in an ideal world you'll be sleeping. But when you've been impacted by an event, or for whatever reason found yourself awake, you can still use it to your advantage. We can learn to accept the reality of being awake and still use the time effectively by resting the mind and body, even if it won't sleep.

I'm definitely not encouraging or endorsing that you stay awake on purpose at night so that you discover the secrets of your soul, because as I'll come on to explain your dreams can do that whilst you're fast asleep. I'm also not recommending you set your alarm for 4am (unless that's when you get up for work). However, if you're awake anyway and can't get back to sleep, it's definitely worth exploring that there may be some helpful answers in the dark.

Whether you resonate as someone I described earlier who feels like being awake in the middle of the night is a waste of time, or find yourself staring at the ceiling, sighing at the unfairness of it all, I am going to suggest your wakefulness can be useful *without* you getting up.

There is something about the stillness of night that can provide a healthy clarity and optimism, once you know how, to understand where you're going and what's stopping you.

It might give you the breathing space to tune in to your mind, body and soul, to appreciate what you need, and what might be missing. Whatever the reason you're awake at night, consider that it holds possibilities – and hope – worth exploring. If you want to, we can take a step further in to darkness in the next chapter, where I'll share my own experience of it.

**Activity:** If you want to, you could continue to use your journal in the morning to record why you think you woke up in the night. Were there thoughts going round your head, or is it possible an external noise (like a door slam) woke you up? If it's happening at the same time every day, is there a practical reason for this? Someone once told me they would wake up every morning at exactly the same time – 4.15am – but only at certain times of year. When we explored it, she discovered that was the time their central heating kicked in. It was the "click" of the heating that was waking them up in the lighter stages of sleep.

# Desiderata
Max Ehrmann, 1927

Go placidly amid the noise and the haste, and remember what peace there may be in silence. As far as possible, without surrender, be on good terms with all persons.

Speak your truth quietly and clearly; and listen to others, even to the dull and the ignorant; they too have their story.

Avoid loud and aggressive persons; they are vexatious to the spirit. If you compare yourself with others, you may become vain or bitter, for always there will be greater and lesser persons than yourself.

Enjoy your achievements as well as your plans. Keep interested in your own career, however humble; it is a real possession in the changing fortunes of time.

Exercise caution in your business affairs, for the world is full of trickery. But let this not blind you to what virtue there is; many persons strive for high ideals, and everywhere life is full of heroism.

Be yourself. Especially do not feign affection. Neither be cynical about love; for in the face of all aridity and disenchantment, it is as perennial as the grass.

Take kindly the counsel of the years, gracefully surrendering the things of youth.

Nurture strength of spirit to shield you in sudden misfortune. But do not distress yourself with dark imaginings. Many fears are born of fatigue and loneliness.

Beyond a wholesome discipline, be gentle with yourself. You are a child of the universe no less than the trees and the stars;

you have a right to be here.

And whether or not it is clear to you, no doubt the universe is unfolding as it should. Therefore be at peace with God, whatever you conceive Him to be. And whatever your labors and aspirations, in the noisy confusion of life, keep peace in your soul. With all its sham, drudgery and broken dreams, it is still a beautiful world. Be cheerful. Strive to be happy.

# Into Darkness

*Only when we are brave enough to explore the darkness will we discover the infinite power of our light.*
~ Brené Brown

Despite the title of this chapter, I'm now *not* going to start talking about *Star Trek*, although I'm a big fan of Benedict Humperdink, as my daughter likes to call him.

This section is actually about exploring our *fear* of the dark.

If we're going to find answers in it, we need first to consider why we're scared of it. Like a lot of things, once you realise there's no longer anything to be afraid of, you feel more confident in dealing with it.

Darkness is not just the absence of light when the sun goes down. It is the implicit suggestion that the opposite of light is something bad. To prefix something with the word dark can be interpreted as something sinister; our language reinforces our fear of it.

Dark side.

Dark humour.

Dark web.

Dark secret.

Even when we talk about mental health, we often describe someone's mood as dark, especially when thoughts are taking them to "a dark place".

They all imply something ominous, or wrong.

I highlighted that the research is fast building a picture of a global sleepless society, but for those of us who do manage to sleep trouble-free during the night we can usually attest that when we wake up refreshed the next day, it was because nothing bad happened overnight. And yet, there is something about the dark.

Darkness can feel as if it takes on a faceless form, an amorphous entity, that roams through the house when light disappears. We can't see it, but we feel like something's there and you're not alone if you're afraid of it.

Fear of the dark goes by many different names, like achluophobia, lygophobia, nyctophobia – specifically, fear of the night – and scotophobia. There are different theories about why we don't like night-time, especially the dark, and it may be rooted in our evolutionary history.

Thousands of years ago, humans were most at risk at night. Back then, we were the hunted, not the hunters. Beasts would prey on us as darkness fell when we were at our most vulnerable, because predatory animals have incredible night vision, whereas us poor humans don't. We weren't safe at night. So, for as long as we've walked the earth, and often unknowingly, we've been programmed since birth to be fearful of the dark. There's research that supports this.

Fifty years ago, psychologist Frederick Snyder first proposed that animals who live in groups stay vigilant whilst asleep. We saw in Myth #3 it was hypothesised that at least one member of the household won't sleep as well as others (if at all), because of an evolutionary "sentinel reflex" to stay awake and keep guard, as David Samson later investigated.

Essentially what this suggests is that a reason you're awake and everyone else is asleep in your household is because *you're* the one feeling responsible for everyone's safety. If you live alone, the same would apply except it's your safety you're understandably looking out for.

In *Tired But Wired*, Ramlakhan goes on to explain:

*… for every human being, there is a very basic and primitive need to feel safe and secure before we can sleep.*

Ramlakhan also describes the need for an "inner core of safety" that remains strong even during adverse times.

If we have blurred boundaries with friends and family, or even reminders about work laying around the bedroom (like a work phone by the bed), these could be what's disrupting our sense of feeling safe, and thereby subconsciously keeping us awake.

One way we might try to counteract this is by leaving a light on in the house.

My earliest memories of bedtime as a child were that we always slept with a light on, usually in the bathroom. The bathroom was directly opposite my bedroom, and next to my mum's. Back then, I believed the light was on in case we needed the loo during the night; the light provided clear passage between rooms, and that made perfect sense.

Today, knowing I grew up in a house filled with superstition and ritual, I'm also confident the bathroom light was a form of talisman, the equivalent of a church gargoyle, to keep evil at a safe distance. Light keeps the darkness at bay.

The darkness can also create chaos when it feels untamed. If you're someone who knows what it's like to have thoughts circling through your mind at night, the darkness feels frenzied, even dangerous, all the while in the outside world everything is calm, quiet and still.

The thing about the dark is that it also amplifies. It can take a feeling – like regret, shame, sadness – and make it seem a thousand times worse (or more).

It can make relationship breakdowns and other painful events feel as if life is just too hard. It can take thoughts – like "what if..." and "if only..." – and make your brain feel like there's an angry, spinning somersaulting beast inside your head. It's like the Tasmanian Devil from the Warner Bros cartoon, but nowhere near as funny. Best case scenario, swirling thoughts at bedtime are like being on the Tea Cups at the Fair. You know it's no fun, you wish you weren't doing it, and realise you can't get off in the middle of it. It's no wonder we wake up feeling sick and tired.

I think it's fair to say that most people are afraid of something, even if they've only been exposed to it once. You might have woken up from a bad dream, or perhaps once were woken in the night with bad news; as a result, the dark becomes the enemy. You become nervous or terrified of it, in case something bad happens again.

For some people the change of seasons (and for example the dark nights) can also contribute to a type of emotional darkness, a consideration like Seasonal Affective Disorder, or S.A.D.; you can find out more about this via websites like Mind.[34] Bright Light Therapy, counselling and medication are just some of the remedies people find helpful, especially where poor sleep is a factor.

We can also inherit our fears through people we look up to or consider to be in authority, or from behaviour we've seen which might give explanations to phobias of events we've never experienced. Your fears may actually be ones your parents or caregivers had growing up.

I once knew someone who was afraid of getting on an escalator. When I asked if they'd ever had a bad experience of one they said no, but that one of their parents was terrified of them. The fear wasn't originally theirs but they carried it with them to keep them safe; children to some extent may learn what they live – or at least find ways to feel safe modelled on how those in their lives with authority behave.

So, if your parents were afraid of the dark even if they didn't explicitly say it, their actions might have, it stands to reason you might be too. In the same way, if they told you that *you* should be afraid of the dark, even in jest – for example, "Don't let the bed bugs bite!" – you'll start to recognise where some of that fear comes from.

It's also important to recognise that darkness isn't always

something we see, but something we feel. But as you'll hopefully see below, that's not necessarily a bad thing.

## The Shadow Effect

*The conflict between who we are and who we want to be is at the core of the human struggle.*
~ Debbie Ford

Within each of us, there is usually a side we don't like to admit, or want the world to see. Nothing sinister: it could be our love for a particular reality TV show, an emotion we hide from others like jealousy, or it could be something we keep literally hidden, like a secret stash of chocolate we don't tell the kids about.

Think of the times you've lost your temper because rage was piling up. Or when you've hidden a like or dislike, in case people thought worse of you for it. We are often brought up to not talk about things that make people uncomfortable, even if there's no reason to hide it. This is how stigma and social taboos thrive.

For a long time, people had to hide their sexuality and could even go to prison for it. This wasn't a "darkness" of their soul, but society made them feel they had to keep out of sight or be locked away, until most of us caught up with the idea that love is love.

The point is, whether it's socially acceptable or not there is usually something about ourselves we don't like and label it under what we might think of or describe as a dark side. Not Darth Vader dark, but nonetheless something we don't want the world to see or know.

Lots of people have written about it.

Debbie Ford co-authored a book with Marianne Williamson and Deepak Chopra calling it *The Shadow Effect*. Sometimes referred to as our shadow side, we are taught not only to be afraid of it, but as I've explained, to hide it too. The good news is, if it's something we've learned we can unlearn it too.

In Charlie Morley's book *Dreaming Through Darkness*, he describes that there are actually two sides to our shadow. The dark side can take the form of our repressed emotions or desires which are often perceived negatively, like anger or thoughts about sex. Our golden shadow, as he describes it, might reflect our talents for example that we hide from the world so as not to be seen as a boast.

Morley explains that until we learn to harness the energy the shadow uses, we will be wasting it in ways that don't serve us well. We *need* to make friends with our own darkness, and allow it to provide the answers we seek.

Most famously, Carl Jung suggested that until we integrate the shadow in to our conscious way of being, we will never feel balanced. Trying to push away our shadows, or pretending they don't exist, not only takes up a lot of energy, but brings the darkness more sharply in to focus.

Over the years, people have shared with me how the moment the light goes out and their head hits the pillow, that's when the darkness really hits. You might have had a relatively good day but the moment it's dark, your brain turns in to an unstoppable machine, producing thought after thought after thought.

People tell me they feel like it's driving them crazy, that they want and need to shut off their minds. They can keep themselves busy all day, not think about a single problem they're faced with, or maybe manage to push it away. But inevitably, the moment the sun goes down it surfaces in the dark.

The dark can also bring us face to face with our fears, frustrations, and overwhelming sadness. And when it feels so intense, we might just want it to stop.

I can relate to this.

CONTENT WARNING: *This remaining part of the chapter includes a personal story which describes thoughts of suicide and talks about domestic abuse. Please look after yourself if you choose to continue reading this section, and reach out to someone who can help if you need. You can skip this part if you want.*

> *Only in the darkness, can you see the stars.*
> ~ Martin Luther King Jr.

One of the biggest myths about suicide is that a person must have shown signs of depression to consider it, when in fact a person may have just reached a point when they've faced knock after knock, or loss after loss, and a single event may trigger a moment of complete overwhelm. They don't want to die, they just don't want to feel pain anymore.

My dad died when I was eighteen, my first marriage ended in divorce five years later, a second pregnancy ended in miscarriage. I then discovered I was in a relationship where I was regularly subjected to violence and abuse. A short while in to that, I found out my partner was cheating. Again.

On that particular occasion I remember collapsing, feeling like I couldn't breathe; someone literally had to come and help me up off the floor.

I don't know how long I was laying there, I just remember the shock and disbelief, and experiencing grief as a physical pain in my body.

I remember bizarrely hoping it must be a sick joke, insisting it couldn't be true, and that life could just go back to "normal".

My thoughts flitted between, "How could he do this to me again?" to me reprimanding myself, asking what could I possibly have done to cause him to behave that way. (That's the At Fault Position – we take responsibility even when we've done nothing wrong.) I know now, I wasn't to blame.

This man was a bully. He was often violent. In fact, he was abusive in every way you can imagine.

But at the time, somehow, all I felt I "should" do was beat myself up.

Although I knew about counselling at that point in my life, I was still working full time for a large organisation but not then as a counsellor. I didn't know much about domestic abuse. I hadn't seen the signs. So I blamed myself. (Even those who are usually good at giving advice, and looking after others, realise they're not always so good at helping themselves. It's why I now practise what I teach, especially about self-care, *every* single day.)

When life deals us a sucker-punch, we resort – often unconsciously – to our go-to coping strategies.

In the past, whenever I have found life too abrasive, I would go to bed. It's one of two coping mechanisms I'd had for a long time – the other being Jaffa Cakes. Before I regularly practised mindfulness and self-compassion as I do now, I would fall in to these unhelpful habit loops that my brain would authorise because I just didn't know any better.

I know for many people, and for different reasons, the bedroom can have negative associations. For me, even with all that happened to me as a victim of domestic abuse when something awful happened, my bedroom was always my sanctuary, my escape.

The problem was on this occasion, I was trying to escape what felt like inescapable feelings, and at that point they were more intense than I'd ever known. Anything I would have told someone else to do in that moment, was somewhere far away in the back of my mind and out of reach.

I've learned now, as I will share with you, that trying to push away pain is usually what amplifies it. As I've highlighted, the very meaning of the word depression is something which has been pushed down.

But at the time, I just wanted to hide from it *all*, to travel in time by way of sleep to a place where I didn't feel this pain anymore. I was lost inside my own head. I felt hopeless.

On that particular day, having discovered I'd been betrayed again, as the night drew in, the darker it became both outside my bedroom and inside my head. It was almost as if a curtain came down, like it does in the theatre to confirm the performance is over. I remember thinking, "I can't go on."

I mentioned earlier that time is often skewed at night; a minute can feel like an hour, or before you know it it's the early hours of the morning. It was still dark outside, and I hadn't slept at all; my mind sounded like a dozen brass bands tuning up inside my head. There was no effable noise, just a thousand thoughts about the unfairness of it all, and who was to blame. That night, I blamed me.

People will carelessly ask why a person doesn't "just" leave an abusive partner, and that's often a sign they don't understand. Abuse isn't always physical; it can be insidious, calculating and leave you questioning your own sanity. People stay because of threats – i.e. to their own safety if they leave, or that of their children or pets. They might be being coerced or controlled, isolated from family and finances. They will question their own state of mind asking "is it me?" I remember thinking how embarrassed I felt for putting up with someone like that for all that time, and then swaying between "what's wrong with me?" and "I just want this to stop."

Circles of thought included:

"What will people think?"

"What will I do now?"

"I'm too old to start again."

It all just felt, so... desperate. And, honestly, at the time I felt it was. I needed a sign.

What happened next, for me, was a miracle. It's one of the reasons I encourage people to hold on, because you just never know what's round the corner: who is thinking of you, and what the darkness will bring. It might be a dream. It might be an idea. It might be a message.

As I lay in my bed, I reached for my phone. It was a reflex action to pick it up, I don't know why I did, or what I was going to do with it. I saw there was a text from my lovely friend Jim.

Jim had moved to Malta years before, where he was now living with his boyfriend, and we'd kept in touch. He used to call me "Mystic Meg", because I always seemed to "know" things about his life before he'd told me, especially if he was going through a hard time. Sometimes I'd dream about him, because I'd get a sense he wasn't okay. We hadn't spoken that day, so it wasn't like Jim knew anything was up or had a reason to message me in the early hours of the morning (Malta is an hour ahead, so it was even later there than it is in the UK). And yet, somehow, Jim knew.

The message said:

*There will always be bumps in the road.*
*Some are bigger than others.*
*But you will get over them.*
*Read this.*

And with that, he sent me a link to *Desiderata*, the iconic poem by Max Ehrmann.

I read the words and then I read them again. Every time I read it, words would spring from the page:

*"You have a right to be here."*

The words spoke to me in a way that is *really* hard to express in writing. It was meaningful. Calming. Spiritual.

Something changed.

A shift.

An awakening.

A knowing that everything would be alright.

I began crying but they were different tears – hopeful tears.

I fell asleep, and when I woke up the next morning the world just felt different. Not fixed. I wasn't healed. But like I could get through this.

Of course the story doesn't end there, and my answers in the dark didn't just look like a message from Jim. It was time spent awake in the middle of the night, in quiet reflection for more days and weeks to come. Dreams that held my fears and hopes. And even moments of inspiration.

I'm not here to say that after devastating news, years of experiencing one loss after another, I skipped off in to the sunset like a woman wearing white in a tampon commercial and the happiest I've ever been.

There was work to be done, but I took the necessary steps to heal from within. The darkness – both literally and emotional – didn't frighten me anymore.

I knew the morning was worth waiting for, especially once I set the intention to focus on my own well-being. I had friends on speed dial I could speak to during the day, or when I didn't want to be a burden, I would contact Samaritans (who can also be reached by email at jo@samaritans.org). I had my own personal therapy and I found my way through all the grief I'd been holding deep inside.

Was it easy? No.

Does it take work? Yes, it does, which I know is hard when you're tired both physically and mentally. But you can find your way, and you *will* get there.

I'm not comparing my pain to anyone's or minimising it. We all have our own tipping points. What bothers or helps one person, won't someone else.

I'm just saying that however bad it feels, lighter days *will* follow.

As Rumi says:

*Be patient when you sit in the dark. The dawn is coming.*

I'm not sure where I'd be now if Jim hadn't messaged me that night, in that darkness. In the midst of all the pain, and the feelings of rejection and abandonment, I needed to know I belonged on this planet. Not *to* anyone, but that I had a right to exist on Earth.

For me, the answer – one answer – came to me in the dark, through the kindness of a friend in the form of prose. It's one of the reasons today I encourage people to find poetry or spoken word that resonates with them for these darker moments. Things that lift you up, not bring you down; that give you hope and comfort, in a world which is more upside down and back to front than ever.

It could be listening to a favourite song, reading inspiring quotes or keeping the number of Samaritans by your bed or in your phone. You can find *your* answer in the dark, whatever is healthy for you.

I encourage people to reach out, to create a well-being plan, which includes details of who to call if the darkness seems too much.

The darkness can feel like it's bringing everything sharply in to focus, when actually it's just our minds gathering pace. I'm not diluting the impact of it; everything can feel intense during the night, and honestly wretched. We can and do feel hopeless, desperate and alone. We can feel an urge to make it go away in ways which are harmful, but my key message is don't feel you have to act on it. Create a positive plan of action, for what you'll do when the dark feels like it's closing in.

Whether it's a fear of external darkness, or whatever we think is lurking inside, we can learn to sit with it in a way that's meaningful. We can use the time awake as an opportunity for helpful reflection. To avoid the unhealthy and destructive nature of feeling like you're trapped inside your own mind.

We know that how we think, about ourselves and others, can impact our mental health, and create a type of darkness that feels disabling. Our thoughts and feelings – all of them – matter, and the more we try to hide them the bigger problems they can create.

This is why understanding the dark, the nightmares we may have or the answers wakefulness brings, can provide learning how to manage our minds at night.

In the sections and activities that follow, I'll be offering how we can manage thoughts helpfully to reduce some of the darkness, whilst also learning how to lean in, in a safe way, to what we feel.

It's okay to have an aspiration that all will be well, and to believe that something wonderful is about to happen.

*The sunrise is hope's daily invitation to come back to life.*
– Glennon Doyle

## Making Friends with the Dark

*There is light to be found, even in the darkest places.*
~ Gabrielle Bernstein

The idea of making friends with the dark might seem terrifying, but often it's our thoughts about the darkness – not darkness itself – that sets our mind in a downward spiral.

If you have a negative relationship with the dark, it makes sense that you'll be scared of it, and that you'll resist it; you'll be nervous about trusting the night with your sleep.

As a child or adult, if the night-time brought physical pain and fear, then these are memories you might wish to explore with a qualified professional in a safe environment. Always talk to your doctor if you're worried about how your childhood experiences are affecting your adult life.

"Unlearning" a fear takes time, but it can start with accepting it's there. It might seem counterintuitive to confront something we're afraid of, but the reality is it's there anyway, whether you give it a name or not. Remember our instincts to stay awake can look like night-time vigilance even if you're the only one in the house, and I'll offer some thoughts later about how to feel safer at night.

## Suggestions

1) If you have a fear of the dark, see if you can learn ways to accept it. You don't need to analyse why, just acknowledge the fear is present. If it's nightmares that have you worried, consider that your dreams may be helpful, once you know what you're dealing with. I've explored the topic more later but offered some example "darkness" dreams that people have next.

2) Create a safe space. Have a routine to check the doors are locked, windows are closed, and add any security measures you're comfortable with. Your bedroom should be your sanctuary, so make sure your environment lends itself to rest and relaxation. I've offered some ideas around this later on too.

3) Avoid "negative press" about the darkness. Unless you know that there's a local danger, don't read or watch anything that's likely to make you scared of the dark, especially just before you go to bed.

4) Try a night light for a while. Bright lights can keep us awake, but a soft light left on in the house might be enough to reassure you.

5) Manage the fear. You could ask your doctor or local well-being service about forms of therapy that might work for you, or consider a mindful way of life to deal with unhelpful thoughts about bedtime. More on this later too.

## Dreams of Darkness

Sometimes people will have a dream which is set in the dark, or at night. There are lots of reasons you might dream it's night-time, but one is that the darkness might reflect how you feel. If you're feeling in a "dark mood" at the time of the dream, this might be why night-time appeared in it.

In some cultures, dreaming of the night can symbolise a *fear* of death (not a prediction); death dreams can look like many things, and I talk more about these after the chapter *Under Grief*.

Dreaming of someone where you can't see their face because it's dark, or can't tell who they are, might mean you don't necessarily need to know their identity (unless you feel you do know them) but pay attention to how they're behaving. If you get a sense you know who it is, but still can't see their face, this might reflect that the person you're dreaming about feels like a stranger to you, or that you think they have something to hide.

Remember darkness in dreams doesn't always have to be a negative though; if you've had some of your best times at night, for example out dancing or with friends, then it could be a reflection of happier times. How you feel in the dream will often hold a clue to what it means, and I'll explore this more in Part III.

## Create Your Well-being (or Crisis) Plan

Having a positive plan of action can be helpful however you're feeling right now. Whether you've had a tough day at work, or life's been challenging lately, take a few moments to answer the questions below:

### Day or Night:

If I feel overwhelmed I will...... (e.g. turn off my phone/have an early night/have a warm bath)

If I need to talk to someone about how I feel, I will call/ text (name)............

If I am worried about myself I will e.g. ring my GP, call a friend, ring Samaritans on 116 123...

If I need cheering up I will e.g. watch a funny movie, call my friend (name)......

If I need to wind down after a busy day, I will e.g. play some calming music, treat myself to....

## Self-Care Check-In

Take a look at the following questions as part of your morning routine:

How does my body feel today?

What does my body need that I can give it right now?

How will I know if I need to rest or relax today?

What helpful words can I give myself that support what I'm trying to achieve?

What boundaries do I need to set today?

People I can call or message if I need to talk today:

..............................................................................................

Things that help put a bit of sparkle in my step:

..............................................................................................

## Evening Check-In

This is something you can try in the evening, perhaps when you get home from work.

I'm feeling the following emotions

..............................................................................................

Are these feelings stored in my body? If so, where.............

(If feeling tense, you could try three deep breaths. With the exhale, imagine tension leaving the body.)

Something kind I can say to myself about today...........

To benefit my health and well-being, I will do the following this evening:

..............................................................................................

If I need help I will

.................................................................................

If you find yourself awake in the middle of the night, you can also do some – if not all – of the above.

## Note to Self

~ Matt Haig, Extract from *Notes on a Nervous Planet*
Keep calm. Keep going. Keep human. Keep pushing.
Keep yearning. Keep perfecting. Keep looking out the window. Keep focus. Keep free. Keep ignoring the trolls. Keep ignoring pop-up ads and pop-up thoughts. Keep risking ridicule. Keep curious. Keep hold of the truth. Keep loving. Keep allowing yourself the human privilege of mistakes. Keep a space that is you and put a fence around it. Keep reading. Keep writing. Keep your phone at arm's length. Keep your head when all about you are losing theirs. Keep breathing. Keep inhaling life itself. Keep remembering where stress can lead.

# Going Down the Plughole

*A ruffled mind makes a restless pillow.*
~ Charlotte Brontë

Thoughts are like hiccups:

They arrive out of nowhere.

They're hard to get rid of, no matter what you do.

And they get annoying after a while; the more you try to suppress them the louder they get.

We can think about everything and anything. You may even be thinking about your own thinking, a term known as metacognition.

It's frequently reported that we have 60,000 to 80,000 thoughts a day[35] with the majority of those being what you thought about yesterday, and a fair proportion of them negative.

Thoughts can be addictive; thinking is not something we can just get up and do without, we have to learn ways to control it. We cannot just stop our minds from having thoughts, but thankfully there are ways to manage them and that's what I'm going to cover from here on in; this can also positively influence our dream content.

We can invest a lot of time and energy in thinking and don't even know we're doing it. We can lose hours of the day lost in thought, many of those thoughts can be unhelpful or unhealthy. We can go round and round (and round) in circles with our thinking, especially at night.

We can tie ourselves in knots.

Turn against ourselves or someone else.

It can literally hurt.

Whether scientists agree or not, it can be argued quite convincingly that whatever you give your time and attention to, you'll get good at it. So just as you'll become skilled at playing the piano the more you practise, the more you worry the better you'll get at worrying.

We might try to push thoughts away for a time. We might succeed in distracting ourselves for a while. But eventually the thoughts return and depending on how toxic they are, they take us down a metaphorical plughole. And it is dark down there.

Going down the plughole could also be described as "rumination" – thoughts which spin around inside your head, but are inevitably not good for you.

They are the ones that don't really go anywhere, might not make any sense, but usually have the effect of feeling like a huge weight pulling you down. They can involve a lot of negative words, self-judgement or blame, beating yourself up, and calling yourself names. Thoughts you've had a hundred times before, circling endlessly, and that won't seem to leave you alone.

Descartes said, "I think, therefore I am." Thinking is something we all do, every one of us – it's literally what makes us human. Even Buddhist monks and nuns with 25 years or 50,000 hours of meditative practice under their metaphorical belt will tell you they still get lost in thought sometimes, and have stuff rolling around in their minds (those I know say it's mostly about what they'll have for tea).

However, when you suffer with anxiety or depression, or know what grief and loss feel like, it's hard to explain to someone who doesn't – or chooses not to understand.

If you experience the signs of what psychiatrists call Obsessive Compulsive Disorder (OCD) for example, you'll know what I mean when I say you have to get a thought "right" or "neutral" before you can carry on about your day.[36] If you've had a bereavement, you'll recognise other people's attempts to cheer you up when you talk about something that you saw or heard today that made you feel sad. (More on this next.)

In reality, if you don't give your mind something healthy

to do – like focusing on a project or hobby, or pausing with mindfulness – it *will* find something to think about: it might be thoughts about whether you're good enough, where your life is going, or when did it all go wrong. And for many of us, this happens a lot in bed.

At night, even when things are going well in your life, you might suddenly recall that argument you had 20 years ago and what you should (or shouldn't) have said, which will keep you awake for at least the next two hours. Sometimes you can't even make out what's rattling around in your mind, something's just annoyingly "there"; someone once described it to me as like listening to a wasp in a jar.

These moments of dysregulated thinking can take you down the plughole, and in to territory that feels overwhelming; we might even wonder if we'll ever find our way back up.

We can experience this when we're feeling frightened or have been triggered by an event. If you're someone who recognises this, and you're awake in the middle of the night, you'll know how dark it can get.

For a long time, scientists believed that the mind and body were two separate considerations. As time has gone on, we now know that the body speaks the mind. In the same way, dreams can speak for both. How you feel in your body, can affect your mind and vice versa.

Does that mean then, with relatively good physical and mental health, can any of us just stop thinking? The short answer is no, but the quality of our thoughts might change.

To clarify, it's not *thinking* that's bad for you – in fact it's natural.

Our mind is designed to think, that's its job.

Without thoughts, we wouldn't stop at the edge of the road to make sure it's safe to cross. We'd put salt in our tea instead of sugar. And life would just be incredibly boring. We would all be walking around like Zombies, not enjoying a single moment because we wouldn't think about *anything*; we wouldn't be able to appreciate the little things, like a piece of music, a sunflower or a warm, woolly jumper on a cold winter's day.

So why does our mind spin off like a pinball machine?

To quote Danny Penman, in a BBC Breakfast interview,[37] who co-authored *Mindfulness: A Practical Guide to Finding Peace in a Frantic World*:

*This is entirely normal. The mind is designed to think so it's hardly surprising when you close your eyes it chases off, like a greyhound after a hare.*

Whether you try to sit down and rest for five minutes, and your brain nags at you about wasting time like I described in Myth #1, or your brain starts whirring the minute your head hits the pillow, that's normal.

I've flagged already that your brain is designed to keep you safe.

It has a complex system of functions and processes finely tuned to ensure your survival, and send the necessary messages which respond to perceived threat and danger.

Our automatic stress response, most commonly known as "fight or flight", is exactly that – automatic. We don't enter in to an overt and conscious discussion with the brain which weighs up whether to release stress hormones or not; it just does, depending on our lifetime of experiences and all the times we felt pain before.

When you burned yourself on the iron or the oven that time, your brain created a virtual red flag which says, "Be careful!" or "Don't do that again, it hurts." So we take more care next time we use those appliances.

But the brain can't tell the difference between physical and emotional pain – all pain is pain – any more than it can tell the difference between a real or perceived threat.

Someone sends you a text message, which they usually put a kiss on, only this time they didn't. What would you think? Adopting the At Fault Position, you might immediately assume "What did I do wrong?" and start to worry about what you do next. Even if 30 seconds later, the kiss arrives because they forgot or were busy, or it got stuck in the ether, your brain has already dumped adrenaline and cortisol in to your body as if the threat was there, and real.

Just as you'll learn to avoid situations which cause an injury, your brain can also steer you away from things that might cause pain emotionally too, especially if you've been hurt before. Here's an example:

If you want to, imagine for a moment, you're going to a five-star restaurant.

Everything about the restaurant is perfect. The food is mouth-wateringly delicious. The venue is stunning. The customer service is excellent. The staff know you by name and seat you at your favourite table. And, to make this even more perfect, you're going out for dinner with the celebrity of your dreams. Now, imagine these perfect evenings go on for days and weeks and months.

Then, for reasons they may or may not explain, your celebrity turns to you over dinner one evening, and says they can't see you anymore. Now, would you go back to the restaurant?

If you instantly answered, "No," you're not alone. It's the answer people usually give when I ask this question in my classes (although some also say it depends how good the food really was).

When I ask people why they wouldn't go back, they explain that although there's nothing wrong with the service, or food, or scenery in this imaginary space, it's the memory of being there, and the associated pain of going back without the person they cared about.

This is an example of the impact of grief which isn't exclusive to the death of a loved one (more on this next).

Even in this imaginary scene, people acknowledge that they wouldn't go back somewhere that might cause them pain. The brain registers pain. It creates red flags. And it's how we end up avoiding people and places, if the memories hurt. Our thoughts affect how we feel, and our feelings can have a direct impact on what we do, and by extension our mental health.

In his book, *A Monk's Guide To Happiness*, Gelong Thubten says there are four main factors that lead to stress:

1) Not getting what we want
2) Getting what we *don't* want
3) Protecting what we have
4) Losing what we love.[38]

All of these, especially losing what we love as this book aims to show, will affect how we sleep, and dream.

But there is no straight, dividing line between "good" and "bad" mental health. If it's a line at all it's a curve that can go up and down at any point, every single day.

We used to think it was poor mental health that stopped us sleeping. But we now know that lack of sleep can cause poor mental health.

Our mental health can be affected by any number of things including our lifestyle, and life-changing events like bereavement, redundancy and divorce. We've already learned (and the Sleep Cycle Repair Kit expands) that making small changes to our daily habits, like cutting down on caffeine or winding down before bed, can set ourselves up for a better night's sleep.

There's more though.

As I've highlighted, when we wake up in the night, it's not that we're awake that causes the problem – it's what we *think* about being awake.

If you're someone who berates or punishes yourself, saying things to yourself like, "I'm awake again, what's *wrong* with me!", you'll probably find you can't sleep even longer; remember, the brain isn't designed to let you sleep when you're stressed.

Instead, if you acknowledge the way the mind works and the fact that you're awake at night, which as we saw in Myth #3 night-time waking is not necessarily anything to worry about, you can honestly say to yourself, "I'm awake, this is natural," and your relationship with sleep can begin to change.

Getting in to a battle with our thoughts – especially a noisy mind tackling worry or grief – can make matters worse. When we learn to accept the struggle – that a thought is just a thought – that it doesn't need our time or attention, we can give ourselves permission to go back to sleep. You don't need to act upon what you think or conclude in the middle of the night; as you've seen, I actively discourage it. The past and the future really only exist as thoughts in our minds, they're not here and now.

In short, don't believe everything you think.

Essentially then, we each have a natural self-defence mechanism which keeps an eye out for danger and threat. The problem is, as we've seen, because it can't tell the difference between a real threat and a perceived one, the brain responds as if a real problem is on the horizon, and the drive for managing safety takes the wheel.

The part of our brain that processes logic and rational thought literally shuts off, creating a fog in our thinking. You'll recognise it when someone asks you a simple question, and all you can answer is, "I can't think straight."

With our logical, rational mind off-line the main reference point we now have is the past. The brain asks itself, "What did we do last time we felt like this?" It looks in the "filing cabinet" of our memory and experiences, and looks for the last, most successful coping strategy. The problem is, these mechanisms can actually do more harm than good.

This is what Dr Guy Meadows refers to in *The Sleep Book* as *amplifiers* – engaging in activities which are meant to help but often don't, and can potentially make things worse.

When your brain perceives a problem – like, "Oh no I'm awake! What if I'm so tired I oversleep tomorrow!" – it has the potential to send your body in to fight or flight. It floods the body with those stress hormones again, and your brain receives the clear message that it's not safe enough to sleep.

Then your brain looks in the "memory bank" and says, "A glass of wine helped you sleep last time," so it authorises another glass of wine before bed. Like most unhealthy coping strategies, over time you find one glass isn't enough and the next you know you've developed a habit or "amplifier", that won't work well in the long-term.

If you always do what you've always done, then you'll always get what you've always got. So, if you want something different from your night-time, you can start with making small – even tiny – changes.

For a long time, therapists have advised that if you can't sleep after 20 minutes, you should get up. There is a basis for this, in that we might then start to see the bedroom as the problem. However, some argue that all this simply does is teach your brain, as it did with the glass of wine, "This is what we do when we find ourselves awake." Getting up becomes the norm, rather than the exception.

It is okay – even preferable – to stay in bed and *rest* if you find yourself awake at night. Unless there's a reason you need to get up (like Granger earlier), or you're becoming so distressed you *need* to move (part of the flight response), you can learn to achieve rest in your place of sanctuary, and notice that a thought is just a thought.

I've spent a lot of time and words focusing on why we can't sleep, and hopefully what I've written so far has helped reassure you that better nights are possible.

I've also explained here how the mind can get in the way, but what if there is an even deeper cause to explore too? In the next chapter, we're going to explore what I believe could be at the root of so much of this, and why an answer in the dark might be something you'd not realised you were going through.

**Activity:** You can start the process of noting if you have dominant thoughts which might be stopping you getting a decent night's sleep. Is there a theme to your thinking at night, is it a situation that's getting in the way, or do you find that your mind just circles in a swirl of noise? Remind yourself that thoughts are just thoughts, and don't need your attention at night. You can give them permission to come back tomorrow if they're helpful.

You can also create a problem-solving worksheet, where you can decide how best to manage whatever it is that stops you sleeping, especially if it's a situation that needs addressing. With your journal, you can then process these thoughts perhaps with the help of a friend, doctor or a counsellor, and come up with useful, healthier alternatives to the way you think about it.

# COVID-19

Now is a good time to remember that grief doesn't just belong to death.

We can grieve for our health. We can grieve for cancelled travel and adventures. We can grieve for lost work and job security.

We can grieve for the effort we put in to projects that will not come to fruition. We can grieve for all the things we were looking forward to which are now on hold.

So let's remember to be kind to each other. Let's be there for each other through our individual losses and in our joint grief.

~ Life. Death. Whatever.[39]

# Under Grief

*Grief, I've learned, is really just love.*
*It's all the love you want to give, but cannot. All that unspent love*
*gathers up in the corners of your eyes, the lump in your throat, and*
*in that hollow part of your chest. Grief is just love with no place*
*to go.*
~ Jamie Anderson

We don't like to talk about death, and we don't like to speak
of dying. At least, we certainly don't like using those words.
I think it's one of the reasons, certainly in the UK, we have so
many other names for it. One can:
Bite the dust.
Pass away.
Cross over the veil.
Or as my mum would say, shuffle off this mortal coil.
We haven't always had a problem talking about death,
but perhaps noticeably over the last century or so it's become
another taboo. With advancements in end-of-life care, at least in
the UK, we've been partially protected from the reality of death
and certainly what it looks like, as less and less people die away
from their own doorstep.

In 2016,[40] almost half (46.9 per cent) of all deaths in England
occurred in hospital, with only a quarter (23.5%) occurring
in people's own home. 21.8 per cent of deaths occurred in
residential and nursing homes, with 5.7 per cent of deaths
recorded in a hospice.

The practical yet humane way in which we might approach
death and dying in the modern world isn't a bad thing, but it
certainly does seem to have changed the narrative. Whilst some
communities around the world recognise that death is part of
life, or the next stage in our journey, in the UK for the most

part we struggle with talking about how it makes us feel, so we generally push it aside.

Where some cultures have specific rights and rituals following the death of a loved one which bring them closer, the conversation about the subject can still feel awkward or uncomfortable to bring up.

For some it feels unlucky to speak of dying. There are those who worry that if they talk about death, it will make theirs happen sooner. Even though we all know we're going to die someday, there's still a nervousness about jinxing it.

It's probably why, according to Which, over 60 per cent of parents don't have a valid will, and 5.4 million people have no idea how to go about making one.[41]

Our general reluctance to talk about it though, and the consequences of that, is probably why the topic of loss is so misunderstood, and has promoted many unhelpful or outdated philosophies about how to care for someone grieving. This includes a model often cited, from fifty-year-old research, which has largely been misinterpreted and suggests grief is ordered and linear.

There are no "stages" of grief.

This is possibly one of the biggest myths of a generation, which simultaneously may have had the most unhelpful impact on society's perceptions of how we care for the bereaved today. The person attributed to saying there were five is not even to blame.

When Elisabeth Kübler-Ross referred to what is now quoted as the most common stages – denial, anger, bargaining, depression, acceptance – she actually hypothesised up to 13 – she was talking about the process of dying, and the importance of end-of-life care. She documented, in her book *On Death and Dying*, what she had observed in patients as they lived out their final days, weeks and months.

She never intended for her important work to be interpreted

the way it has been today, or for it to be applied so generically across so many other areas of work. It was never meant to suggest that grief is as straightforward as walking a line, with a simple beginning and an end.

As her son Ken Ross said:

*The five stages are meant to be a loose framework – they're not some sort of recipe or a ladder for conquering grief... She just wanted to begin the conversation.*[42]

Kübler-Ross included "hope" as one of the stages, but you rarely see this taught in the discussions around supporting the bereaved, or in magazine articles that refer to her research. And as her son suggested, it was never her intention to suggest grief was resolved by viewing it as a fixed and rigid model.

When someone we love dies, we don't pass through a door marked "anger" with "denial" firmly slammed shut behind, purposefully marching towards the plaque of "acceptance", never to revisit those feelings again. Grief is not like that.

It's not one emotion, it's all of them and it's none of them, and we can feel it all at the same time. They don't come in any order, definitely not in stages, and a lot of what you feel, albeit unexpected, might be common amongst the bereaved.

People have told me how they initially felt shame for feeling relieved that their loved one is no longer in pain. Others describe a natural jealousy, when a colleague told them of plans to celebrate a big birthday with their mum, because the grieving person whose mother had just died will never get the chance to do that again.

These feelings can be puzzling, haphazard, and not make any sense at all, especially if the society in which we live won't acknowledge death, or makes it socially unacceptable to talk about how we feel when it happens.

But grief is normal. And *all* grief is valid.

Rather than being linear, grief is more like a roller coaster than it is a flight of stairs.

It is not a one-way street.

It's not a phase.

It is not a to-do list. It's not something you wake up in the morning and say, "Right, that's grieving done. What's next?"

Society's misperceptions of grief make us ill-equipped to cope with it.

The At Fault Position I've talked so much about, combined with the idea that we grieve in a linear fashion, might have us believe we're getting grief "wrong". This is especially the case if friends or colleagues suggest to us that we should be further down the line than we are, when someone we cherish has died.

And that's another thing.

The inability to have meaningful conversations about the subject of death and dying also means that friends, colleagues and family say the most unhelpful things when you're already going through a difficult time.

Anyone who has ever felt loss – which as I'll explain is not just physical death – will know of well-meaning individuals who at some point have said something like "it's time to move on".

But, the truth is, you don't "get over" grief.

You go under it.

It's a weight that sits on top of you, and slowly you find your way towards the surface again. But at any given moment, a song could come on the radio, or you see something they would have loved for their birthday, and you find yourself under it again.

Society's expectation that someone will be "over it" simply within a matter of days, weeks or even months is shocking when you think about it, and yet this perception is very, very real.

You only have to look at organisational Compassionate Leave policies in the UK (most of which offer between three days and two weeks off) to see the perception that grief is something you do over a short period of time – as if it's like having the flu – and then you're fine.

Even worse, society punishes – even vilifies – people if they need more time off work than policy dictates, as if they "should" have "moved on" in their grief by then.

In my time working with the bereaved, I've heard of many situations where people were subject to disciplinary procedures, because they needed time off to help cope with different scenarios relating to the death of a loved one. Because the organisation rates performance by the number of absences an employee has in a year – regardless of reason – they were penalised for it and put on a "performance plan".

Society – another amorphous entity by the way, with no face but a *very* loud voice – has an opinion on grief, and for what you can grieve. The unhelpful conclusion is you must be doing something wrong if you haven't "moved on", are still talking about it, or feeling the effects of it, a few weeks down the road. The assumption is, you just fix it or snap out of it. It's the outdated "cheer up/chin up – it could be worse!" philosophy, even though things really are as bad as they look.

You'll know already how comments come in thick and fast when you tell someone you've had a bereavement. Friends and associates can say some of the most outrageous things, usually starting with the words "At least...", in their efforts to help you look for a silver lining.

I know of one gentleman, whose wife died not long after the COVID outbreak, who had a friend tell him, "At least now you can pay off your mortgage." As Brené Brown beautifully said: "Rarely, if ever, does empathy start with the words 'at least'."

It can cut like a knife when people try to cheer you up out of grief, and can actually do more harm than good; what you hear the other person saying, albeit implicitly, is "this is making me uncomfortable, please stop talking about it".

Megan Devine, in her exceptional book titled *It's OK That You're Not OK* writes:

*People offer suggestions for how to get out of your grief faster. They tell you what they would do if they were in your position. They tell you about their own losses, as though every grief is exactly the same... Even without comparison, words of comfort from other people can still feel horribly wrong... If you cringe or feel angry when friends or family try to comfort you, it's because you hear that second half of that sentence, even if they don't say it out loud. The implication is always there, speaking louder in its own silence: "stop feeling how you feel."*

You've probably noticed when you go to someone with the news that something bad has happened, their response is to go in to problem-solving mode, sometimes known as the Fixing Reflex.

It's with good intentions, they want to make you feel better, and to take your pain away; we can probably all admit we've been guilty of this at some point in our lives. But the truth is, we know it doesn't really help when someone's grieving.

It's one thing if your child comes home and tells you there's a problem at school, or your friend or partner needs your advice about a situation at work. You can offer an opinion, and work together to figure something out. However, you can't put a plaster on grief, or apply a one-size-fits-all solution.

Years ago, following the death of a close relative, a lady (we'll call her Alice) told me about the time, in the midst of her grief, she turned to one of her friends and asked rhetorically, "How long am I going to feel like this?" It's a reasonable question, and Alice wanted her friend to reassure her along the lines of, "What you're feeling is normal, it's okay if it takes as long as it takes. I'm here for you."

Instead, because of the human tendency to seek solutions, Alice's friend's immediate reaction was to go home and Google that very question. The next day, her friend came back to Alice, excitedly, to report her findings.

Miraculously, Google had come up with two answers.

"The first theory," Alice's friend said, "is that it will be a month for every year you knew each other." Seeing Alice's perplexed reaction, the friend continued, "Or it will be a year, and a day." (Needless to say, this didn't help Alice either.)

When I tell this story at my workshops, every grieving person understands this reference to a year and a day. They know friends and colleagues who have tried to reassure them that once you've had the first birthday, the first Mother's Day, the first Christmas, and the anniversary of their death, "you'll feel better". As if you'll wake up on day 366, all mended, and whisper to yourself, "Wow, that was a rough year."

But the reality is, the second year can be the hardest, and not because the pain is more intense, or the feelings just as raw. It's because no one says a word.

The friends don't call to say, "I know it would have been their birthday today, how are you doing?"

The cards stop coming.

The text messages dry up.

The assumption is you've moved on; that you're "over it".

As Nora McInerny says in her powerful TED Talk,[43] following the death of her husband, Aaron, four years earlier:

*I haven't moved on, and I hate that phrase so much and I understand why other people do, because what it says is that Aaron's life and death and love are just moments that I can leave behind me and that I probably should... We need to remember that a grieving person is going to laugh again and smile again. If they're lucky, they'll even find love again. That absolutely, they're going to move forward, but that doesn't mean that they've moved on.*

So how does this all fit in to sleep and dreams, and why have I written a whole chapter on grief, and the subject itself weaved into and throughout this book?

When you're lying in bed at night and can't sleep, there's a reason. It might not be obvious straight away what that is, but there is one.

We explored earlier (and will do more in The Sleep Cycle Repair Kit) what you do during the day can affect how well you sleep at night. But there might be something else.

You might not have thought of it like this, but the reason you're awake at night might be that you're under grief.

In all the years I've been working with people, whether they've come to me because of problems with work, their partner has left or they just want to get their sparkle back after a difficult time in their life, they often realise they're grieving, or afraid of losing something or someone they love.

The trouble is, society doesn't recognise it as that. This is largely because of our societal perceptions around what loss is and what we are given permission to grieve for.

## What is loss?

You can suffer a loss when anything that mattered to you is no longer there, and as a result of that loss you can experience grief. People will concede that loss can take the shape of a relationship breakdown or redundancy, but don't always connect that what they are going through is the same grief they would experience if someone had died.

Here are just some examples of why people grieve, without anybody dying:

| Redundancy or Retirement | Receiving a promotion |
|---|---|
| Moving Home | Changing School |
| Having a baby | Not being able to have a baby |
| Menopause | Failing an Exam |
| Illness or Injury | Being a Victim of a Crime |

These events can be devastating, certainly difficult for some, but because not everyone recognises what they're going through is grief, they don't know how to manage it, or feel they can't legitimately talk about it. And if they do, they think – or are given the impression – that there is then a time limit on how long they can feel that way or talk about it, and so their grief goes underground.

Grief can live where you might not think it does. It can help to unpack this a little more, with an example.

When Nara was working for a large company, she sat in an open plan office and, over time, became great friends with the people around her. At 11 o'clock each morning someone would come round with the tea tray and they'd make each other a brew. Until she got promoted.

Nara was moved to an office on her own, on the floor above. Not only did no one come round with the tea tray anymore (you might think that's minor, but I promise it's not), and neither did they talk to her. She had gone from being their peer to their manager, and they didn't know what they could or couldn't say, or if she could be trusted. (I hear this story all the time not just in the private sector, but especially amongst police officers working their way through the ranks.) Incidentally not only had she undergone a loss, but so had they.

When Nara tried to talk to someone senior about it, they dismissed and minimised her feelings with comments like she "should be grateful" or she'd "made her bed so she should lie in it." No one understood the loss she was feeling, and so she stopped talking about it. Nara then developed problems sleeping, and when she did sleep she would have some really troubling dreams. (You can see some example loss dreams in the next section.)

Just to show how common this is, when I give this example in my classes, I often see people give each other knowing looks that they've either felt that same way as Nara, or they've said that "should" to someone else. I've seen colleagues nudge each other on workshops, and pull a face of "Eek".

On one occasion during the break, I asked two of the attendees I'd seen pull an "Eek" face, what they'd taken from that discussion. They explained that a colleague of theirs had come up to them only that week, having recently received a promotion, and said that he was finding it hard being away from his team. I thanked them for sharing and asked them how they had responded to him.

They said: "We told him he should get on with it, and that he should be happy he's had a promotion." They told me, following our conversation, they were going to ring him during the break, and see what they could do to help. They hadn't seen his potential grief until we'd talked about it, because it didn't "look" like grief in the traditional sense.

When I describe loss in this way, people will challenge me that you can't compare the loss of a job, for example, to the loss of a loved one, and they'd be absolutely right; we should never compare one experience of loss to someone else's.

However, we must take time to understand that all grief is valid. If I don't understand your loss, and say something unhelpful to you, your grief may have nowhere else to go but inside; this can negatively impact a person's mental health.

When we create a hierarchy of grief – a general belief that there are some things you can grieve for, and some you can't (or that you're allowed to feel sad for a while but not too long) – this can create problems where a person might not feel seen or heard.

Society might think it's "fine" for someone to grieve for the death of their grandparent for example, but not their cousin. I've seen and heard about Compassionate Leave policies that only allow for the death of a "close relative", i.e. mother/father/ grandparent or child. But what if their cousin was like a brother or a sister?

We might think it's ridiculous for someone to be distraught

when they lose their mobile, for example, but then understand a little when we learn there were photos of someone they cared about on that phone that they'll never get back.

If you're looking sad because a relative has died, your neighbour might be okay with it (unless it's a few months down the line in which case they might tell you "it's time to move on"). But tell them you're sad because your rabbit just died, and they might say, "It's only an animal." When someone shows such little sympathy in this way it's called disenfranchised grief.

Disenfranchised grief is when society doesn't recognise or acknowledge that you have a reasonable reason to grieve, and so you feel unable to mourn publicly. For a long time pets were seen as "just animals", although today it is slowly becoming more widely accepted that they're part of the family.

However, disenfranchised grief can take many forms and another's inability to recognise it can cause real problems for the person going through it, especially if they weren't allowed to talk about it. The impact of this can take its toll on how well we sleep, what we dream, and ultimately our mental health.

Disenfranchised grief is a relative and subjective experience.[44] Examples people have told me about include:

- the person who had a miscarriage in the first few weeks of pregnancy and was told, "At least it wasn't a real baby yet,"
- a termination of pregnancy where the person was told, "Well it was your choice,"
- a lady whose family didn't accept her sexuality and when her wife died was told by them, "At least now you can have a 'proper' relationship,"
- the veteran who has lost a limb,
- or the assumption that autistic people for example don't feel sad (or anything at all), because they might display emotion differently.

These generalisations are so unhelpful to a grieving person. It puts them in metaphorical boxes about for what and how they should grieve. And so they just stop talking about it.

Disenfranchised grief doesn't just affect an individual, it can affect an entire community and even go worldwide.

When Take That went their separate ways, a hotline was set up to support their fans; the potential impact of the band's break-up was recognised. But because no one had died, it was mocked by many. When Princess Diana died, despite the outpouring of grief seen globally, I met many people who said they "didn't get it", almost sneering at those who mourned. But that doesn't mean the grief – felt individually and as a nation – wasn't valid.

Princess Diana may have been a symbol of struggle or hope that many could connect with. Or perhaps those grieving knew what it was like to lose their mum, and her death gave them permission to grieve. On the band, the last time someone had gone to a Take That concert, it might have been with their dad who's no longer alive. Their first Take That CD could have been bought by their nan, who died just a few months ago. It may have been a connection to the music, and an acknowledgement that there will never be another song written by that group, where they felt they belonged. Music gives many people purpose, and is a form of therapy. It makes sense that they grieve for it when it's taken away.

I would almost bet you a Jaffa Cake that you can remember where you were the day you heard a famous celebrity had died. If we just take musicians, whether it was Freddie Mercury, Prince, David Bowie, George Michael or Chester Bennington, lead singer of Linkin Park, you can admit to me if you shed a few tears.

But I'll also wager if you did show your grief at the time, there were others who didn't understand why, and maybe even called you a "snowflake" or similar, if you did. Labels like "snowflake" are derailing, and so stigmatising, and usually feel like they shut the conversation down.

This is what disenfranchised grief looks like. It halts a conversation that really needs to be had. And when a person doesn't receive the response they need, they will tuck their grief away.

In the same way if you're scared of losing someone or something, that may become an anxiety. Anticipatory grief is the feelings of grief experienced *before* someone dies, but is experienced as if the person has already gone.

This has been felt acutely during COVID, where there has been a raised anxiety that those we love will die, especially if they suffer with pre-existing medical conditions.

In the same way as we can go in to "fight or flight" even when the perceived threat isn't there, when we are afraid of loss it can affect us as if it's happening too.

When grief has nowhere to go, it goes underground. Sometimes this might take the shape of a constant stomach ache or muscle pain that can't be explained by doctors – sometimes known as inhibited grief.[45] Even anger may be hiding as or driven by a primary concern of fear, or loss (of control).

If you've had an experience of loss which has remained unresolved or is "incomplete" in your journey through life so far, either because you weren't allowed to talk about it or because you didn't realise that's what it was, then it may well have had an impact on how you sleep and how you dream.

*Nod to Grief Research: Time is* not *in fact the great healer. Through his studies, Dr Robert Neimeyer discovered it is not the passage of time that helps someone heal, but making sense of their loss;[46] how a person spends their time grieving.*

*One of Worden's Four Tasks of Mourning: is to "work through the pain and grief". However, it's important to remember that working through that pain should be done at your pace; don't let others dictate how long that should take or how you should be grieving. If your grief feels "stuck", and you've developed unhealthy coping strategies, speak to your doctor or a counsellor who can help.*

# Dreaming about Death

*Where you used to be, there is a hole in the world, which I find myself constantly walking around in the daytime, and falling in at night.*
~ Edna St. Vincent Millay

This is a category of dreams that understandably upsets people, and is often one that people ask about for help.

I've taken the opportunity to explore this here as I've been talking about death and dying, and its relationship to sleep and dreams. I've also included some other anxiety dreams later in Part III, where I will also offer how you can start to work with your own dreams in a meaningful way.

When the news broke about COVID-19 and that it had become a global pandemic, the subject of death and dying came sharply into focus. We saw – and at the time of writing are still seeing – heartbreaking daily updates of who has died in our region, country and across the world.

As a direct result of the virus, we know that dream recall is up 35% and, according to the Lyon Neuroscience Centre, people are having more negative dreams. If you've been having dreams of death since the outbreak, this might explain why.

However, dreaming of death is not a new thing, and earliest records date back to Ancient Egyptian times. The Chester Beatty Papyrus 3, discovered at Deir el-Medina, dates back to the 19th dynasty (1220 BCE) and is an example of ancient dream exploration.[47] It talks about death, and is believed to contain a reference that suggests if a man dreams of having sex with a woman, he will experience a period of mourning.[48]

Of course we know now, thousands of years later, that far from being a prediction of death and dying, death dreams are more likely a representation of change. This will hopefully come as a great relief to anyone having sex dreams which, again, are less likely to be literal and instead interpreted as about connection, power or control. I want to take a moment here, on a serious note, to highlight that dreams of this nature – whether about sex or death – can be distressing or disturbing and may be the echo of an actual event that happened, where the details appear in the dream as they were in waking life.

Where this is the case, and particularly if these dreams may be a sign of trauma, it's always important to speak to a professional so they can offer help as soon as possible. There are links to organisations that might be able to help at the back.

Whilst culturally death in dreams will mean different things for each community, they can recognise that we – and those we care about – transform and change as time passes. When we notice how rapidly things – and people – can evolve in our lives, it makes sense this sits underneath our conscious awareness for a while. As our priorities change, our focus shifts, life adapts.

House moves, children leaving home, redundancy, retirement and ageing can all bring about a dream of death; not because it's imminent or predictive, but because the "old" life is no longer there. Dreams of being lost can happen at this time too.

This explains one reason for the increase in our dream recall, as we navigate a global crisis and see changes around the world. *Everything* is transforming – from the reduced number of cars on the roads, to aeroplanes in our skies – even how much food and toilet roll was on the shelves. The emphasis has been on lack, loss – including freedom of movement – and literally in everyday conversation on death itself.

It makes sense that we process this awareness of change as an ending, and it symbolically plays out as death in a dream.

It can also reflect our *fear* of death, especially when we are seeing it in the news every day. That's why you're just as likely to dream of dying during a pandemic, as you would be if you embarked on a journey of personal growth.

Death in dreams can also represent noticing change in other people, including our children and parents as they get older.

When the level of care we provide for a child changes as they grow up, we might subconsciously process this as our input in their lives has finished (even though it hasn't). When they leave home for example, our brains might translate that as the death of the relationship, even though in reality it might be the connection between you has just transformed into something new, and they're probably still very much available at the other end of the phone.

In the same way, if a parent or loved one is coming to the end of their life, this can be a constant thought at the front of your mind which plays out in a dream at night. Your dream may be trying to prepare you or help you process what's happening and search for ways to cope with the news, especially if you feel you can't talk about it during the day.

All these things can have an impact on why we dream about death itself, as an echo of a fear or worry.

They are distressing but dreams about dying are common, especially at a time when death is in the daily conversation. It's understandable then to dream about losing people we love, *because* we care and don't want them to die.

It's natural to worry someone you love will leave – physically or emotionally – and this anxiety can also manifest in our dreams. A common dream people have is their partner is cheating, but that doesn't mean it's happening or going to come true; the most likely reason is the *fear* of that event. This is why it helps to talk about what you think and feel, so that it doesn't manifest in your dreams at night. (I have covered this in more detail in Part III.)

Let's say for example, in your waking life, you're noticing something different about a person you care about; their behaviour, their looks or their outlook on life has changed. This can be symbolised by dreaming of their death, because that relationship is currently under the spotlight. It's not that they're going to die, but the person you want them to be has gone.

It is also a common dream for parents to have, as children get older. It's not a reflection that something bad is going to happen, but most likely because the parent is seeing some sort of change in their child.

To dream of losing children is common at particular stages of their lives, especially when they're toddlers and again as they grow into their teenage years. This may well be because, at these ages, you start to notice a change in them, in that they're less likely to "need" you on a practical level. The death in the dream therefore can represent their transition into adulthood, and our emotional response to that; losing what they once were to how they now are – associated with feelings of redundancy or rejection, but symbolised as loss or death.

## Dreams of Causing Death

The messages around Coronavirus have put the responsibility of others' safety in our hands with the slogan "Save Lives"; if you dream you have inadvertently caused the death of someone, this might explain why.

It's not common for it to be anyone's intention to pass on the virus, but a dream that you did could be an acknowledgement of the fear and concern about how the virus can be spread. Dreams often echo our fears and frustrations like that.

If you dream you have killed someone, this can symbolise the pain or hurt you may – or fear you may – have caused them, and the worry this has damaged the relationship. We sometimes say "well that's killed it" meaning that we've potentially brought about the end of something, albeit unintentionally.

I spoke to a lady who told me she'd been having dreams lately that she stabbed her partner. They were in a committed relationship and she was lost as to why she'd dream about doing something so violent and far from her mind. I asked her if she worried she might have hurt him lately, and she nodded. She said that some weeks before, during an argument, she had lashed out and said something really unkind; he'd said at the time it was like a "knife to his heart". Although they had made up, and she'd apologised for what she'd said at the time, she was still feeling guilty about it.

The act of killing in the dream could also be a metaphor for something ending – if for example you dreamt you were killing a beast, the monster could represent fears that you're learning to control.

If someone is trying to kill you in the dream, this may symbolise the hurt someone or something is causing you. We sometimes say, "This is killing me," especially when we talk about work or a relationship. If the person hurting you in the dream is doing the same in your waking life, then it's essential to get help as soon as it's safe to do so. There's a list of agencies in the back that can hopefully help.

In essence, it's important to explore who and what is dying in your dreams – and how – and seeing if this relates to fears and worries you have in your daily life.

## Types of "Loss" Dream

*Answers in the Dark* is not a dream dictionary and it's not possible – or helpful – to speak in definitive terms, so rather than say what every dream might mean there is a section later that offers some ideas about how to interpret the dreams you are having. The following are just some of the common grief and loss dreams people have, including when no one has died. Remember that everyone is different, and dreams will always depend on the context and circumstances:

- Feeling lost, can't find your way home, can't find your car or can't find a parking space. This is common if you're not sure where you "fit in" at the moment, especially after retirement as well as the death of a loved one.

- Taking a journey to or from somewhere, and particularly when you miss a plane, train or bus. Many people describe waiting on a platform and not knowing when the next one will come along. One explanation can be a metaphor for a lost opportunity (e.g. "I missed the bus") or the journey of life and the challenges and frustrations it presents.
- A house or a home, possibly one you grew up in or spent time in at a significant point in your life. This could reflect that you're missing a different time or place, or that something happening now reminds you of something that happened back then. People bereaved by murder may dream their home has been invaded.
- Trees in dreams can reflect the Tree of Life, as well as how we think of the strength of a person. For example, you might have a dream that a tree falls down after the death of a loved one, the tree representing the one you love – the fallen. In the same way, we might have death dreams in the winter, because everything in nature looks like it's dying, even though it's waiting to be reborn.
- Losing teeth is one of the most common dreams that people have globally, and it's fascinating how the interpretation of this can vary across cultures. In some communities to dream of losing teeth is a warning (not a prediction) that something bad may happen (like the death of a loved one), whereas in many cases it represents the fear of loss itself. In the UK and in the US, we have a tradition where, as children, we exchange teeth for money. So a dream of losing teeth might represent a fear of losing our status or wealth. I will say though, if you've watched the TV advert where the person brushes their teeth and then spits out blood in the sink, you might well go to bed that night and dream your teeth fell out *if* you're literally worried that might happen.

- Falling can be common after redundancy and bereavement, because it can reflect that feeling of not knowing what's going to happen next, a bit like Alice falling down the rabbit hole. It's not to be confused with the hypnic jerk or myoclonus – a "twitch" that occurs as you're dropping off to sleep. There are lots of reasons we have these (for example hiccups are another type) but one theory is that it can be a symptom of how stressed you are (stored tension in the body being "shaken off" at night), or it might just be how you're built. Chat to your doctor if they stop you sleeping well.

- Bumblebees, robins and feathers are sometimes considered to be "messengers" from those we've loved and lost, but again this depends very much on what you were raised to believe. I'm conscious that in some cultures for example black cats are lucky, when in others they're not. (I'll talk more about how to unpack symbols later.) One common theme since Coronavirus has been that people are dreaming more of insects. The loose translation of this could be, from a metaphorical point of view, that insects are bugs, and they can spread disease; if our brain has processed COVID-19 that way it would explain why people are having that dream.

- Chasing or being chased in a dream is another common one which has many possible translations that extend beyond the subject of death and dying. However, some people do have this dream when their intense emotions are "catching up" with them from grief (in the same way that some might dream of tidal waves), they need to "catch up" with some work, or they feel they've been left behind. Catching the virus (or a fear of catching it) might be another interpretation if you're the one being chased.

- Bridges in dreams can be fascinating symbolically (Freud was said to have made all sorts of assumptions about these), however, in the context of bereavement, it can represent the space between you and your loved one who is "on the other side". One common dream is that a grieving person will see their loved one over the bridge but can't get to them, reflecting the fact that they're now physically out of reach.

- Standing on a shore can be similar to the bridge dream after the death of a loved one, as it can reflect the distance between you and someone who has died. Water in itself has many meanings, but in the context of grief often symbolises the strength of emotion we might feel. If the water is calm for example, this can suggest you're coping okay.

- As strange as it may sound when a partner dies, you may dream they are cheating on you, death being the "person" that stole your loved one away. It can also be a fear of loss. I talk more about this later under *Anxiety Dreams*.

- Kisses are a bit like sex dreams, in that they're not often about what you might think. For example, they can be a symbol, especially after loss, that you want someone to forgive you (or vice versa); the kiss being a symbol of making peace with someone else.

## Visitation Dreams

When you dream that someone you've loved and lost visits you in a dream it can be a special and transformative moment – these are sometimes called Visitation Dreams. People I've spoken with who have had this type of dream say they wake up feeling settled, reassured and that they can take a step further forward along the road to healing.

Some people never dream about their loved one again, even though they wish they did. However, it can also be particularly unsettling if the person who has died behaves in a way that is unkind or unexpected in the dream. This can particularly be the case when bereaved by murder or suicide.

When this happens, it can be helpful to explore whether you feel there is any "unfinished business" or unresolved thoughts and feelings, perhaps a conversation you wish you'd had.

People often feel guilty for many reasons – even though they don't need to – after the death of a loved one, mostly about things they wish were said or done prior to the passing. Some feel they should have done more however impossible this may have been. That's the thing about guilt, you don't have to have done anything wrong to feel it.

Sometimes in a dream, people will appear to "snub" you – i.e. you try to talk to them but they ignore you and don't reply. In the same way, when you try to talk you can't speak or you can't hear what they're saying. Whilst this might acknowledge they are no longer here, it may also represent a concern now they're gone they can no longer hear you.

Some communities believe that dreams are a way to communicate with the deceased, and many cultures around the world consider dreaming as a way of receiving helpful messages from their ancestors. Dreams of this nature are usually seen as a pathway to enlightenment in some way – the content is never unkind or hurtful – but instead provides valuable information for the dreamer to take positive action in some area of their life. People who have healthy visitation dreams often wake up feeling as if something really magical has just happened.

Having worked in this field for so long, I feel confident in saying dreams where deceased loved ones appear in a way which is unkind or hurts you are more likely reflecting a worry, regret or concern you have about their passing. If they tell you in the dream it's time for you to be with them for example, consider this may be more a reflection of the depth of your grief, and time to reach out to someone local for help.

Bereavement is rarely straightforward and dream content during the grieving process can seem cruel, even years after the person has died. But it is important to allow yourself time to understand the impact of loss, how you're dealing with their death and consider how this is reflected in both your waking reality and dream life. Talking things through with a close friend or a professional can be a helpful place to start. Ironically, the more we push our emotional pain away during the day the more it might show up in our dreams at night in the form of a nightmare.

A note on nightmares: I'll talk more about these in Part III but remember dreams are offering you the chance to explore what's really on your mind. If your dreams are disturbing to the point that they're making you ill, please talk to someone.

## Managing Grief

Whilst I could write a whole book on the different ways in which people grieve, just as I won't tell a person definitively what their dream means (only offer food for thought as I've done above, and explore), it's not possible to write a "one-size-fits-all" philosophy on what helps manage feelings of grief. The journey takes as long as it takes, finding your way at your own pace ideally without "Society" telling you how you "should" be doing it. However, I've included below some things which people have said they've found helpful over the years.

- Being able to talk about the loved one, especially with people who remember them.
- Keeping a memories box, which contains keepsakes that represent what was most special about that person. This could contain anything that prompts a fond memory, from an ornament, a photo album, a birthday card or a bow tie.
- Planting a tree in memory of a loved one, or commemorating a favourite place they'd visit with a bench or plaque. During the Coronavirus outbreak, we also saw yellow

hearts placed in windows in remembrance of someone who died of COVID-19.[49]

- Writing a journal or letter. Some people find this therapeutic, and you can write to yourself or the person who has gone. (This may work just as well for any loss, as it does for someone who has died.) You can include significant statements such as "I thank you for... I'm sorry for... I forgive you for...". I recommend if you do this, to ask a friend to be on standby just in case it brings up a lot of emotions. You don't have to keep the letter, you could keep it in the memories box, or destroy it when the time is right.

- Remembering to eat, get fresh air and stay connected. Finding people who understand grief can be a big help (see below). And don't feel you have to rush grief.

- People who come together in either a formal or informal setting can provide support to each other, and share their hopes and concerns about death and dying. One example is the establishment of "Death Cafés" > https://deathcafe.com.

## How to Help Someone Grieving

I've included this in case you're caring for someone grieving right now, and aren't sure how to help. It's important not to tell someone how they should grieve, and the most helpful things bereaved people say you can do is listen and be there for them, as often as you reasonably can.

Try not to shift the conversation on to you, e.g. by telling them how you felt when someone died or when something bad happened to you; it can feel like a comparison (or at worst, a competition) and won't necessarily offer the support they need right now.

Put your phone down when you're holding space with them, and if you can't visit, check in on them regularly even if they say, "I'm fine."

If you feel you want to do something helpful, you could ask if they need practical support, like cooking a meal or walking their dog.

Signpost to suitable organisations if you're really worried or ask them how they'd feel about having a chat with their doctor.

Take care of yourself too, so that you can help when needed.

*What NOT to say to someone grieving –*
When I offer the following to people in training, sometimes they cringe in the knowledge that they've said something like this at some point or another. Don't worry, we've probably all done it, and with good intentions. (It's one thing if the bereaved person says the following – you can take your lead from there – but try not to say it first if it's meant as a "silver lining".) These are some of the things to keep in mind going forward, that people have (genuinely) told me they wished others hadn't said:

x They wouldn't want you to be upset.
x I think you might be wallowing.
x They're happier where they are now.
x Be grateful for what you had.
x You're still young, you can always have another child/get remarried.
x They had a good innings.
x I know exactly how you feel.
x You need to take up a hobby/make new friends/do yoga/ eat avocado.
x Don't you think it's time you stopped crying?
x At least you still have your health (or any sentence that starts "At least...").

Whether you're someone who is grieving or with someone else who is, a key thing to remember is that it's how we spend our time in loss that can affect how we cope. The kindness of others matters, whether it's a week after the event, or remembered two years down the line. Be kind to yourself in grief, and reach out for help when you need it.

## A Grieving Society

I started this book explaining that we are now a Sleepless Society. But from the work I've been doing in the last two decades, I also believe we're largely a grieving one – for the loves we've lost, the chances we feel we missed and the life changes we've faced. Because we're discouraged from talking about their impact it makes sense that our fears, frustrations and experiences show up in our dreams and through poor sleep It's my belief that sleep, dreams and grief are all connected, noticeably since the arrival of a global pandemic. By now you've hopefully also seen that if you've experienced loss in whatever form that was, that might be what's getting in the way of both a good night's sleep, and how well you dream. Whether you identify with loss or not though, I've pulled together a Sleep Cycle Repair Kit next, along with a whole section on dreams for you to explore.

Embrace your grief, for there your soul will grow.
– Carl Jung

## "Some Very British Problems with Sleep"

~ Rob Temple (@soverybritish), *Born to be Mild*
1. Trying to get to sleep while also thinking about that time when you were nine and said a word wrong and the whole class laughed.
2. Being horrified to find out that you've been sleeping with the buttoned-up end of the duvet on the side.
3. Telling someone about your elaborate dream in which

loads of cool stuff happened and... oh, look, they've walked away.

4. Remembering with fondness the days when a lie-in meant staying in bed until 2pm rather than 6.15am.

5. Hearing a knock at the front door while you're still in bed and thinking that being very, very quiet will somehow make it all go away.

# Part II

# The Sleep Cycle Repair Kit

Up until now, I've focused on the *why* of poor sleep, and how it can affect our dream content.

Essentially, I believe grief that is hidden or stored away – either because it's unrecognised or repressed, where a person has not had permission to show it – plays a large part. It's not the only reason we don't sleep but the hundreds of people I've worked with have said it makes sense in their own personal journey of discovery. Shining a light on grief can help take some of the darkness away.

In this section, we're going to recap and explore the nature of sleep, and consider how to manage the mind when it feels like it's acting up, so that you might eventually be able to make friends with night-time (or hopefully at least not dread it). It's not "repairing" your sleep cycle as such, more like a recalibration or finding your way back to it.

Sleep isn't something you just switch off and on, in the same way that dreams are not just the subconscious rattling of the mind. There is a reason why we can't sleep, and there is a reason we dream what we do. The following pages will explore and offer tips on what might help.

I've called this a Sleep Cycle Repair Kit, but of course it's not a band aid that you put over something, or a problem that can necessarily be mended overnight. I often say, "If you always do what you've always done, you will always get what you've always got." Like everything in life, healthy change comes with small moments of progress that happen with understanding, effort and commitment, and a willingness to be curious and explore what's really going on. I'm going to revisit some of what I've already offered and expand where it might help. Let's start with how you can tell if you're not getting enough sleep.

## Early Warning Signs

- have trouble focusing or can't concentrate
- forgetful
- can't make decisions (especially "good" decisions)
- feel sleepy, especially when it's inconvenient (like in that meeting just after lunch, where you nod off just as someone asks you a question)
- feel sick and/or hungry for sweet things
- gain weight/can't lose weight, even when you try to diet
- feel edgy or get easily irritated
- burst in to tears but not really sure why
- yawn a lot
- don't feel refreshed when you wake up, like you still need more sleep
- have slower reflexes and reaction times
- seem to get every cold and bug going round
- fall asleep watching TV

These are just some of the "early warning signs" of sleep deprivation – a few are milder than others. Signs of extreme lack of sleep can include hallucinations, paranoia, and blurred vision. If you recognise these latter warning signs, get an appointment with your doctor as soon as possible.

## The Functions of Sleep

Sleep is believed to hold a number of important functions, including the repair of our physical body and maintaining the health of our minds. We sleep in stages and, for the purposes of this book I've divided them in to three, categorising them as light sleep, deep sleep and Rapid Eye Movement (REM) sleep.

Specialists in sleep science theorise more stages than this, or categorise them in to REM and Non-REM (NREM) but I want to keep this simple. There are many books on the science of sleep itself if you want to dive a little deeper; I've referenced some in this book already.

I said before that sleep is not like a switch you simply turn on and off. You are never always in deep sleep, just as you're not always in light sleep and, paradoxically, brains can be awake and asleep at the same time.[50] We transition through each stage, throughout the night, many times.

We cannot do without sleep. If it was enough just to rest, then we'd do that without ever feeling the need to go to bed. However, rest matters and I will come on to explain how you can do that effectively when you just can't seem to doze off.

I likened the arrival of sleep earlier as similar to a bus route which can help you to know roughly when it will arrive and determine the best time to go to bed: i.e. when you're sleepy.

Some people have told me they can sleep anywhere, anytime – but if you're someone who can't, you will definitely know what it feels like to be laying awake, waiting for sleep to come. (Incidentally, being able to sleep anywhere, anytime can also be a sign of sleep deprivation, so chat to your doctor if your sleep doesn't refresh you especially if you could fall asleep standing up.)

I liken sleep then to a journey, and it has a specific route. Every night we plan to take that ride, but for one reason or another it can be disappointing, or doesn't turn out the way we'd hope. It is a trip we are meant to take though, whether we want to or not.

In our sleep, we travel in to a world we are not generally consciously aware of, and as we surrender to the adventure we can visit faraway places, see things we've never seen and meet people we've never met, through our dreams.

In an ideal world, we will start the journey at night and make it several times before waking, each journey taking an hour and a half or so, the approximate length of our sleep cycle.

As explored earlier, the human body is cyclic by nature.

As well as our sleep cycle, humans have at least:

- a 24 hour cycle: day follows night, follows day
- a 365/366 day cycle: we label as a year
- a 28 day cycle for those of us who have a significant period of our lives (pun intended) where we can usually expect that too.

If we're observing these rhythms and honouring their patterns, our body has more chance of working efficiently, functioning like a series of beautifully timed systems that work harmoniously in sync with each other. If you've ever watched *The Big Bang Theory*, this is probably how Sheldon Cooper is able to set his watch by his bowel movements, as a rather random example. If you go to sleep later than usual, you might find your bathroom schedule is off the next day too (as well as when you eat, of course).

We also know the human brain *loves* routine; it helps it – us – feel safe.

The brain wants to know – *needs* to know – what's going on, so that it can plan and prevent; so it can connect and control.

We are born with an automatic pilot which develops over time, freeing up more space for you to think instead of do. All of this is done for our benefit, to ensure our survival. However, while it learns as it lives, if left unchecked it can learn to see danger *everywhere*.

Your brain is always responding to your environment in one way or another. In the search for sleep it's generally looking for whether it's light or dark, how noisy or quiet, and ultimately if it's safe. When the brain interprets that the circumstances are right, amongst other things, it produces melatonin. This slowly increases during the evening, and starts to decrease as morning approaches. As it begins to kick in, you might start to feel sleepy.

Each sleep cycle has a rough length and a destination, which follows a specific route, which is why I use the bus analogy. Each stage can be identified by different brain waves, which is where the electroencephalograph, or EEG, came in handy for trying to determine what we're doing at each particular level of sleep, and what influenced decades of Dement's work. (I'm keeping this explanation deliberately non-technical where possible, largely because I have to type words like electroencephalograph *really* slowly, and if you're someone who just wants to know how to get a better night's sleep, or make the most of your dreams, I don't want to bore you.)

Each stage of sleep is believed to have its own purpose, and I will outline that briefly. Remember that sleep theory is changing all the time, so what we know about sleep today may change tomorrow, just as what we knew yesterday may be different today.

Using my bus analogy, sleep stages are like the roads along your personal bus route. Each road you navigate takes a certain amount of time to travel. When the route's complete, it will start all over again until your alarm goes off, or between 5am and 7am, when melatonin levels may be decreasing.

Let's take a look at each stop along the bus route, or each stage as I've described them:

- light sleep
- deep sleep and
- REM sleep.

**Light sleep** is effectively the start of your journey in to sleep, and also the sign it's coming to an end. It can last 20-30 minutes (ish). This route can be particularly useful if you need an afternoon nap, where you'll "get off the bus" before you head in to deep sleep. (See *The Power of Naps*.)

This is when you may experience what's known as the "hypnic jerk" I mentioned earlier, when you might "twitch" yourself awake as if you've stepped off a kerb you didn't see, or missed the bottom step at home when you're awake. Light sleep is generally when you're dozing off, and as you're waking up.

**Deep sleep** is believed to be largely for restoring and repairing functions in the body. It's understood that deep sleep may be necessary for many things, but one in particular is keeping our immune system healthy.

The body creates a virtual to-do list of things it can only effectively do whilst we're asleep; helping to control weight is one of them. When the body is sleep-deprived, the level of ghrelin spikes, while the level of leptin falls, leading to an increase in hunger.[51] So as well as being responsible for our immune system, not getting enough sleep can lead to things like weight gain too.

Healing the body is thought to be one of sleep's greatest benefits, which I'm sure is one of the reasons we use the phrase "sleep is the best medicine", and perhaps why we have the urge to go to bed when we have a cold or flu.

Lack of sleep may be one of the reasons why, when you've been working really hard and then take two weeks leave, you might feel ill the moment you arrive on holiday. Making sleep a priority is a healthy goal, quite literally.

Deep sleep is longer, and can be around 45 minutes (ish), depending on what time of night it is and the individual length of your cycle. If you try to get off the bus in the middle of deep sleep (for example by setting an alarm for an hour after you dozed off), you might suffer with what's known as sleep inertia – also called "The Hangover Effect". You wake up shaking, with a banging headache and don't know what year it is.

**Rapid Eye Movement (REM) sleep** is the stage we most commonly associate with dreaming. I'm going to talk a lot more about this in Part III but from the science-y perspective, it's given its name by the way our eyes move quickly from side to side when we are sleeping, which usually indicates a person is having a dream.

Everyone dreams, even those who say they don't, with even babies spending a fair chunk of time in the womb doing so. Scientists are starting to suggest that we actually can dream in any stage of sleep, but those that happen in REM sleep are the ones we tend to remember, if we remember them at all.

Incidentally, if you set your alarm to wake up during this stage of sleep, you're more likely to remember your dream. In fact, some people even find if they fall back to sleep at this point, they'll go right back in to the dream they were having. That's great if you were dreaming something lovely, not so much if it was a nightmare.

One area I touched on earlier which can help with sleep was Sleep Hygiene, and I'll expand more on that here.

## Sleep Hygiene

This is the name given to what you do during the day and in to the evening, that can affect how well you sleep.

We all develop habits in life and those that shape our routine (like washing our hands) can be important, especially when we're navigating our way through a global crisis.

However, sometimes these habits can have a longer-term effect, which over time becomes part of the problem, especially if those habits produce changes in the body (like stimulants for example) that can prevent us from feeling sleepy when we need.

Changes to your habits and routines don't have to be huge, and certainly don't have to cost you any money. It's why I encourage people to start with small daily changes and build from there. You don't need to have much motivation or willpower at all to make a change in your life or reach a goal, you just need to make the activity small enough that it's easily within reach.

I'll expand on this shortly in the context of sleep, but if you want to learn more on how to make or break a habit, you might like the TED Talks I've referenced by Judson Brewer[52] and by BJ Fogg.[53]

The key is recognising what's not helping and then doing something different to what you've done before. There are practical things you can reasonably do every day that might improve how well you sleep at night. Below is an example of a sleep hygiene questionnaire which I was given during my training with permission to reproduce that can help determine what habits you might need to make or break.

*Example Sleep Hygiene Questionnaire*
Anything that's outside the "good" column is worth looking at for change. I've offered some suggestions underneath.

|  |  | GOOD |  |
| --- | --- | --- | --- |
| 1. Do you go to bed/wake up at the same time every day? |  | YES | NO |
| 2. Do you drink a lot of tea/coffee/caffeinated drinks? | YES | NO |  |
| 3. Do you smoke, especially just before bedtime? | YES | NO |  |
| 4. Do you have a "night cap" to help you sleep? | YES | NO |  |
| 5. Do you have a heavy meal after 8.30pm? | YES | NO |  |
| 6. Do you make time to unwind before bedtime? |  | YES | NO |
| 7. Do you keep yourself busy well into the evening? | YES | NO |  |
| 8. Do you check your mobile phone in bed? | YES | NO |  |
| 9. Do you go to bed when drowsy? |  | YES | NO |
| 10. Is your bed comfortable? |  | YES | NO |
| 11. Is your bedroom quiet, secure, dark and cool? |  | YES | NO |
| 12. Have you spoken to your doctor about sleep problems? |  | YES | NO |

## Sleep Hygiene Top Tips

#1: Go to bed/wake up roughly at the same time every day, aligned with when you feel sleepy and naturally awake. The reason we say this is because as I've suggested your brain loves routine. If you vary your bedtime too widely (e.g. more than half an hour each way), you'll find it harder to sleep and it can knock everything else out of sync. It might sound like a drag but try to keep to this routine every day, even on a weekend. If you tend to lay in you can suffer with Social Jet Lag, explained more later.

#2, #3, #4: Avoid stimulants before bedtime. Caffeine, sugar, nicotine and alcohol can get in the way of a good night's sleep. When people ask me what time of day they should stop drinking coffee, I usually say about three days ago; depending on how sensitive you are to caffeine the effects of it could stay in your body for days, not hours. Try to cut back, especially after lunch. (If you drink a *lot* of coffee, alcohol, or are a heavy smoker, don't just stop. Manage the withdrawal safely, ask your doctor or a support service for help.) Although you might think that a "night cap" helps you sleep, as it wears off and the alcohol metabolises in to sugar it might wake you up. It's why when you've had a heavy session of drinking, you'll bounce in and out of sleep all night. There's also a difference between being asleep and being unconscious.

#5: Don't eat too late. Eating a heavy meal before bedtime can sit uncomfortably and make you feel restless at night. Try to eat a bit earlier so that it gives you time to digest. You can have snacks before bedtime if you tend to wake up hungry, but preferably not anything that's too sugary.

#6, #7, #8: Make time to unwind. TVs and mobile phones are a barrier to sleep in the 21st Century. The light that comes off both can keep us awake, and even devices with "blue light filters" might still trick the brain into thinking it's daylight. Checking your phone in the middle of the night might be enough to make your brain think it's time to get up, especially if it suppresses melatonin, largely responsible for making us feel sleepy. If you give your kids an iPad to keep them busy before bedtime, keep in mind that if light from it affects you, it's affecting them too.

Make the time before bed a place of peace and calm, this is sometimes known as "The Golden Hour" or the One Hour Rule and I'll expand more on that soon.

Dim the lights, put on some calming music in the background, have a warm milky drink and read something that's not too exciting and easily forgotten (this applies to children *and* adults). Avoid watching the news, checking social media, or responding to emails. Deal with your "to-dos" long before you think about sleep.

#9: Go to bed when you're sleepy. I've talked about this at length already, but this really is a key ingredient for getting a better night's sleep. If it's practical and possible, go to bed when your eyes feel heavy.

#10: Get a comfy bed. I've expanded on this below as well too, but you'd be surprised how many people think that because they've only recently bought a mattress, they have to keep it for eight years just because the manufacturer says that's how long it will last. If you can, always try before you buy.

#11: Again I've expanded on bedroom environment below, but one top tip I'll give here is to make your bedroom a "No Whinge / Argument Free Zone". Energy lingers, it's how you can tell when you walk in to a room where there's been a row even if no one's talking. Keep your bedroom somewhere that's calm and peaceful, that lends itself to healthy vibes. If you do have a whinge zone in the house, make it the garden. That way, you'll think twice about how much you want to argue if you have to stand out in the rain.

#12: I do keep saying it, but it's because it matters, your doctor really is the first port of call if you're noticing significant sleep problems. They might offer a range of options to help, and if they don't, seek a second opinion. In the UK we have an organisation called Healthwatch who, if you're not getting the service you need, can advocate on your behalf.

### Which is better, Lark or Owl?

Some in the field of sleep use terms like "larks" to define those who are up with the dawn chorus, and "owls" for those who might prefer to come to bed nearer midnight. In years gone by, I also used to use these tags when describing groups of sleepers.

However, these days I try not to lump people in together this way; the reason is, because it can give people the impression one type is "good" and one is "bad". Society loves putting people in boxes, and whilst it can be helpful to know when you're likely to feel drowsy, suggesting people are boring if they go to bed early, or a party animal because they like it late, can give people the impression that at least one of those is wrong. In the past, I've even had people ask me how they can *change* from being a lark to an owl, because their partner is the opposite.

I also know that in this day and age, more and more people don't necessarily get to choose when they sleep. they work shifts, regularly cut across different time zones (at least pre-COVID), or for all types of reasons, can't get to bed at the same time every night. So from my perspective it's more helpful to meet people where they are, focus and accept what you can and can't reasonably change, and go from there.

It's why I focus on achieving quality sleep rather than *how much* you think you should be getting, suggesting we replace what *time* you go to bed instead with when you feel sleepy, to improve your chances of getting a better night's kip. If for example you have a bed partner who snores, or works different shifts to you, it's absolutely fine to sleep in another room on occasions so you or they can catch up. People sometimes worry that not sleeping in the same bed can damage a relationship, but if you've ever slept with a snorer, you'll know that actually sleeping in the same room as one creates tensions of its own.

## The Power of Naps

There's been a lot of debate about naps over time. At one time, power naps were frowned upon, either because you were seen as lazy, or the reasonable worry it might impact how well you sleep at night. However, as Catherine de Lange writes in her article "How to Nap Like a Pro":

*Napping isn't lazy – it's a smart way to reap the rewards of sleep.*[54]

Many people say they can benefit from a power nap in the afternoon, if their work or home life supports that. The key to a "good" power nap is the length of time you sleep for.

De Lange goes on to explain:

*A nano-nap, lasting just 10 minutes, can boost alertness, concentration and attention for as much as 4 hours. Take 20 minutes and you increase your powers of memory and recall, too.*

Because we know the light part of your sleep journey lasts about 20-30 minutes before you head in to deep sleep, this has been suggested as the optimum length of a power nap.

However, if you can sleep for longer and it doesn't affect your sleep at night, you might decide to fit in a complete cycle of around 90 minutes to two hours without an alarm – especially if you work shifts. As well as helping you feel refreshed, not using an alarm in the afternoon could give you some insight as to how long *your* personal sleep cycle is.

Knowing about the sleep cycle in this way can help maximise the quality of sleep, and even make organising your day easier. If you know roughly when you'll feel sleepy and when you'll wake up naturally (unless you need an alarm for work) you can plan your life around it. If you know you need to be awake at 6.30am but naturally wake up at 5.30am, it might be better to get up then than lie in for another hour and wake up with the Hangover Effect: groggy and with a fuzzy head. (See also *Social Jet Lag*.)

As we've seen, going to bed at roughly the same time and getting up each day can help keep those natural rhythms in a healthy flow. In fact, not following that rhythm, for example if we tend to lay in at the weekends, may actually put a spanner in the works.

## Social Jet Lag

This is the term sometimes used to describe feelings of grogginess that occur when we're not following the natural rhythms of our bodies, or breaking patterns in our day-to-day lives.

Rather than the disruption to sleep caused by shifting time zones when travelling abroad, we can experience something very similar just staying at home – called social jet lag.[55] When we disrupt our routines by having late nights and early mornings, it's bound to catch up with us in the same way it would if we were making long distance trips across the equator. Here's an example:

Yeraz's alarm wakes him up at 7am every morning to go to work, Monday to Friday, but likes to lay in on the weekend perhaps until 10am, especially if he's had a late night the night before. When he does this, at the weekends, he finds he has really weird dreams, which sometimes startle him awake. When it comes to Monday, Yeraz sets his alarm for 7am but finds he doesn't sleep well the night before, and says he literally has to drag himself out of bed on Monday morning. (See also *Sunday Night Syndrome.*)

Your brain and body work like a series of clocks which sync and work together (this might be why some people say they can "set the clock" by certain things like when they need the loo or when their period is due).

By changing his weekend routine, Yeraz has disrupted the rhythms he'd established Monday to Friday, so that when he goes to bed on Sunday night his sleep is disturbed. As his body takes the weekend to establish the new wake time of 10am, come Monday when the alarm goes off at 7am, Yeraz has to wrench himself out of bed.

As your sleep journey progresses throughout the night, you also have less deep sleep and more REM. This means that although you're staying in bed for longer, you're more likely to spend more time dreaming, than you are getting any more significant rest. It's one of the reasons why many people will say they have some real corkers of dreams when they have a Sunday morning lay in, and explain the increased dream recall since the pandemic began.

*Nod to Shift Workers: For a few years now, I've delivered workshops for police officers, paramedics and search and rescue teams who tell me that shifts are the one thing that plays absolute havoc with their sleep.*

*Whoever you work for, if your job requires shift work, you can probably relate to this disruption, especially in your cycles; those who menstruate may find their periods are irregular or painful. There has been some research[56] to suggest that shift work – and therefore delayed sleep – can have a significant impact on menstruation.*

*My top tips would be to make the most of your rest days, even if you can't sleep, scheduling some time out for yourself to sit and "be". (Some of the meditation activities later may help.) Consider effective power napping as I described earlier, especially if you're going from a set of earlies on to lates. Speak to your boss, company or union about what strategies they can offer, including keeping the lights low at night where possible (especially towards the end of your shift) and periodically changing your shift pattern to more sociable hours when you can. If you're going through the menopause and that's also impacting your sleep, there should be organisational guidance to help with that. If you feel sleepy when you get home but would normally have food first, it's okay to go to sleep and eat later, unless it's the hunger that keeps you awake.*

## Sunday Night Syndrome

If you work Monday to Friday, you might have noticed there's something about Sunday – or for shift workers, the night before you go back to work.

The day may start off well, enjoying some well-deserved rest and relaxation, or catching up on chores, or spending time with loved ones. But early evening, you might notice a shift in your mood – that Back-to-Work feeling.

You might recognise it when your stomach rolls when you think about work, or you even feel a sense of dread. All this can lead to a bad night's sleep.

Sometimes known as Sunday Night Syndrome (or as *Stylist* magazine called it the Sunday Scaries[57]) it can apply to people working split shifts too, whether it's four on, four off, or earlies and lates. Essentially it's "the-night-before-you-go-back-to-work" effect.

Even if you love your job, you might still notice that Sunday or "the night before" brings with it a sense of uncertainty.

We will explore more shortly what helps us sleep and dream better, but thinking has a lot to do with it, as does technology. I remember one police officer telling me they would check their emails the night before an early turn, just to "get in front" of the working week, and then tell me, they almost always instantly regret it.

So, if you're someone who finds that Sunday night – or the day before you start your next shift – gets in the way of your sleep, for some ideas on how to improve sleep more generally, here's some more things which might help:

1) Acknowledge you're thinking. Thoughts and feelings keep us awake; we also know that bottled-up emotions can lead to burnout.[58] As soon as you notice thoughts swirling round your head, or feelings affecting your ability to sleep, acknowledge they're there. Some people think it's counterintuitive to put the spotlight on feelings, but the reality is they're there anyway, whether you notice them and give them a name, or not.

Once you know what's going on in your mind using mindful awareness, you can then manage your mind in a positive way. We'll talk more about this in the section on mindfulness.

2) Talk about it. If work is getting in the way of you sleeping well, it's important you let the people that matter know. Lack

of sleep could be what's affecting your performance, as well as have an impact on your physical and mental health. It's important to nip it in the bud especially if you find yourself in front of the boss having to explain why you're late, or asleep at your desk.

Tell your manager what's on your mind and what is contributing towards it, and see if they can help you come up with a plan that takes some of the anxiety away. If they're not receptive, speak to HR, ask to speak to Occupational Health, or contact your Employee Assistance Programme if you have one.

Talk to family if they're interrupting your sleep if you're working shifts, or if you decide to take a power nap. See your doctor if feelings or worries are getting in the way of your health and well-being.

3) Spend time during the day meaningfully. If you're not already active, the benefits of exercise – and certainly movement – have long been recognised as being able to facilitate better sleep, as well as being good for your body and mind. Go for a stroll during the day, or enjoy some time in nature; a morning walk between 8am and midday might set you up for better sleep at night. Don't leave going to the gym too late in the day though, as exercise too close to bedtime can leave you feeling pumped, and unable to doze off.

Alternatively, maximise a power nap like I described earlier.

4) Turn your to-dos into Ta-Dahs! Write up your lists of things to do during the day, so that your mind isn't racing at night once you've got into bed. If you have to check your emails (which I don't recommend) then do it earlier in the day, rather than just before bed. Keep a pen and paper by your bed if you need to, so you can jot down anything that comes to mind and then leave it until the morning. This works the same for dreams, as long as scribbling in bed doesn't disturb your bed partner if you have one.

Having a routine can also help. Don't forget, we know

having a consistent go to bed and get up routine can prevent Social Jet Lag which can otherwise affect how refreshed you feel next working day.

5) And relax... There are lots of ways you can prepare yourself for the week ahead, and set yourself up for a good night's sleep. I've described good sleep hygiene already and we'll have a look at mindfulness too, which has been proven to help people sleep better. Switch off your mobile phone (or at least turn off notifications) and run yourself a nice bath, or find what works for you that's healthy and do more of it. And remember, whatever the week might throw at you, you can handle it.

In the days before the Coronavirus outbreak, we had the freedom to travel wherever we wanted including distant (and local) shores, whether it was on a well-deserved holiday or for much-needed business. However, you may have also noticed that the first night you stay anywhere new, you just don't sleep that well.

## The First Night Effect

If you've ever booked yourself in to a nice hotel, the very least you'd expect is a decent night's sleep. However, the chances are you'll have an unsettled night – maybe even nightmares – at least for the first evening and perhaps for the couple that follow. But why is this?

Some health professionals believe this is partly due to our brain being concerned primarily with our survival. In times when our ancestors lived in nature, and threats to safety very real, unfamiliar environments kept us on "alert" so that in the event an attack was imminent, we would be able to rouse from sleep easily and get ready to either fight or run away to safety. Research by Yuka Sasaki[59] and colleagues seems to support this, documenting what has become known as the "First Night Effect" (FNE).

Essentially, the study suggests that the brain creates another "night watch" in order to protect the sleeper, this time when they're in a new environment. Even a nice hotel room doesn't guarantee us a good night's sleep if our brain is working hard to keep us safe if we do doze off.

Staying somewhere else might also cause an experience where in lighter sleep a person might sense an "entity" in the room, sometimes also with a feeling of pressure on the chest. This has a name.

## "Old Hag" Syndrome

This is a phenomenon where, upon waking, a person feels like they can't move, senses a malevolent presence, only to find there was no one there. Once called "Old Hag Syndrome", this describes a type of sleep paralysis, accompanied by a feeling of pressure, usually on the chest. Whilst it's only temporary, it can be terrifying.

In *States of Mind*, an exhibition by the Wellcome Collection (2016), the curator Emily Sargent wrote:

*During normal sleep the body is paralysed to prevent the sleeper from acting out their dreams. This paralysis is usually released when the sleeper awakes. In sleep paralysis, this release doesn't happen at the right time. Regaining consciousness, the person finds they cannot move and feel a crushing sensation in their chest... In addition, powerful and often unpleasant sensations can accompany an attack, including auditory and visual hallucinations.*

Sargent went on to explain that while the phenomenon still remains largely misunderstood, folklore around the world has provided frameworks of understanding these terrifying night-time experiences for centuries. For a long time sleep paralysis was seen as a sign of witchcraft, or the evil "incubus" – a disturbing nightmare induced by a demon.

In modern-day terms though, this type of "shadow" could simply be trying to tell you that you're stressed or that you're not feeling safe in the environment where you sleep. This is what makes learning to unwind before bedtime so important.

## Hearing Your Name at Night

Another night-time experience that can frighten people awake is hearing their name being called, even though there's no one there. I've experienced this myself, and was intrigued to know if others did too. One time I heard a loud, female Irish voice calling my name (I am a quarter Irish myself but with no living Irish relatives) which woke me up. The voice simply said my name, nothing else, and it woke me up. I wasn't scared, just wondered what it was about and how common. (I will admit, I did take a moment to look around my bedroom half asleep – that's how real it was – but nevertheless no one was there.)

When I first set up my website on the topic of dreams, this was one of the most popular pages visited by people literally all around the world. Although it seems quite common, this type of experience can be unsettling when it feels so real.

The reality is, we *all* hear voices to some extent.

The voice in your head that says it's time to start dinner, or you need to leave to catch your bus, is one you've lived with all your life. You might not acknowledge it as a voice as such, more just part of the thinking process.

As you sit with this book in your hand, you might hear your own voice reading it. When you're missing someone's voice, you might be able to bring to mind something lovely they said, and hear their voice in your mind just the way they'd say it. Perhaps you can call to mind a famous actor with a distinguishable voice, like Michael Caine saying, "You're only supposed to blow the bloody doors off!" You might even wake up, as I often do, hearing a favourite song, as if the singer – and their entire band – is inside your head. (More on that next.)

In his book, *The Voices Within*, Charles Fernyhough normalises these voices, talking about the history and science of how we talk to ourselves. He says:

*Talking to yourself in your head is an ordinary activity... The assumption that voices are always a sign of severe mental illness is a limiting and damaging one.*[60]

Interestingly, in the same book, Fernyhough describes an individual with early hearing loss who described hearing a voice in their dreams.

One theory, of why we hear a voice whilst asleep, is that it happens when we are dozing off in to what's called the hypnogogic state, or the hypnopompic state as we wake up. As this happens, we may have a "voice hearing experience" as a sign that our brain is starting the journey into sleep.

Another is as we transition into non-REM sleep, we may have an auditory hallucination, combined with a visual one, like the ones I alluded to earlier when you think you've stepped off a kerb and jolt yourself awake (the hypnic jerk). Whilst this doesn't necessarily explain why it's our name (or a random Irish voice like I heard), it is a sign that more research in to sleep phenomena is important; the more we know, the less likely we are to be nervous about it.

People who hear their name in the night often want reassurance that nothing sinister is taking place – don't forget, even though I know this is normal, I still looked round the room to make sure no one was there.

Some people have asked me if it's someone they love reaching out, others find it terrifying, especially if it's accompanied with a feeling of a presence in the room like I described in the case of "Old Hag Syndrome" earlier.

There are cultures and traditions today that still believe dreams are a divine portal, for messengers from another time and place to introduce themselves. Some have described them to me as a "guardian" or guide, who brings helpful messages to them in their dreams.

Sometimes the voice can feel calming and reassuring – even angelic. There are many references to dreams in historical texts, like the Bible.

In Genesis 31:11, Jacob had been involved in an unhealthy "to-and-fro" with his father-in-law, where Jacob was being tricked (or taken advantage of, at least). He then hears his name being called, and replies, "Here I am"; with that, an angel appears. The angel suggests enough is enough, that Jacob needs to end the drama, and walk away.

In her book of the same name, Oriah suggests "The Call" is a sign of an awakening, that we are being called "home" – not to a specific place, but to who we truly are. It's asking us to wake up to the world around us, and be authentically true to ourselves. She writes:

*I have heard it all my life. A voice calling a name I recognised as my own. Sometimes it comes as a soft-bellied whisper. Sometimes it holds an edge of urgency... What you are looking for is right here. Open the fist clenched in wanting and see what you already hold in your hand.*

We still don't know enough about this phenomenon to say categorically why it happens, not least of all because of the different ways people experience it. So when people ask me why it's happened to them, I suggest the activity I've included next, and let them decide the reasons behind it for themselves.

If you are someone who has this experience and can't get back to sleep, it might only be because it freaked you out – i.e. not because something bad is about to happen – so knowing how to calm the mind when it's stressed can help.

This is where prioritising feelings of safety at home, alongside normalising certain night-time experiences, can help you get back to sleep if you need.

Having said this, if the voice is disturbing, it's important you speak to someone you trust about it as soon as possible. If it's malevolent or, as can happen in dreams during grief, if the voice is being unkind to you, or trying to tell you to hurt yourself or someone else, it's a sign you might be struggling with all that's going on. Seek medical help immediately so that you can get the support you need. As I'll explain more, dreams are your friends; they would never tell you to do something which would harm you or anyone else.

If you've ever woken up from sleep hearing a song in your head, we'll cover that after this activity.

*Hearing Your Name Activity*
This is where keeping a journal can be useful so that you can start to spot any patterns in your night-time experiences, which can then easily be explained away. You might find you hear your name being called at night when you're stressed, or overtired. Only do this activity if it feels right and safe for you.

Here are some things to think about:

- What gender do you identify with the voice, and is that significant?
- Do you recognise the voice?
- Was the voice helpful?
- How did you feel when you heard the voice?

Deciding how you felt is just as important as why it happened. If it felt like it happened in a dream, and the voice sounded familiar (even if you couldn't see their face) it may be that someone during the day has been trying to get your attention but, for whatever reason, you've not been taking any notice. Hearing the voice at night can "wake you up" to the fact someone – including you – is trying to be heard. Ask yourself who that might be.

If you woke up hearing your name, and you're intrigued as I was, you could maybe say, as Jacob did, "Here I am," and see if the next dream you have gives you any more insight.

If you want to receive specific insights from your dreams, I'll explain more in the next section, but essentially, you could try asking before you next go to sleep – and only if you feel safe and ready to do so – ask to "meet" the person behind the voice in your dreams. It's entirely up to you how you proceed with it; if you're under the care of a mental health team talk it through with them first, so you can do what feels safe and healthy for you.

## Waking Up with a Song

If you've ever woken up with a tune going round your head you're not alone. It's so common, researchers have tried to understand why it might be.

It would make sense if it's a favourite track you're enjoying right now, that you've maybe been playing on repeat. But what about the random songs you haven't heard in years like *Strobe Light* from the B-52's, *She Blinded Me with Science* by Thomas Dolby or a song from as far back as during the Second World War?

There could be a number of different reasons why we get what's known as "sticky music", "stuck song syndrome" or an "ear worm", which might explain why we have a song on our lips when we wake up first thing. Here are some possible explanations.

1) Music Exposure. One explanation is that it's an echo of a song you heard during the previous day or before you went to bed. At the time of writing, whilst navigating our way through lockdown in the UK, we also commemorated 75 years since Victory in Europe day.

As the nation went to sleep singing *We'll Meet Again*, people described how they woke up singing it the next morning. On the

9th May 2020, the English actor, comedian and writer Stephen
Fry tweeted:

*Well, you can't deny that* We'll Meet Again *is one heck of an ear
worm. I went to bed humming it and there it was in my head this
morning when I woke up. I expect it'll leave me but... don't know
where, don't know when...*

2) The Association of Ideas. When someone starts talking about
sleep or feeling tired, you might find that before long you start
yawning. This can be referred to as the Association of Ideas.
When we hear or see something, we register it in our minds,
search for comparisons or mirror it with something similar from
our own experiences.

As Dr Vicky Williamson, a memory expert at Goldsmith's
College London, found from her research, if you shop somewhere
like Faith, your "memory goes down a line of dominoes" until it
reaches George Michael's song of the same name.[61]

It might be then, the dream you've had the night before
triggers a similar domino effect if the song you have on waking
aligns with the dominating thought (from the dream) in your
mind.

3) The Impact of Stress. Williamson goes on to explain, if
there was a song playing when you were revising for exams
at school, then it follows that when you feel stressed you start
singing or "hearing" that song.

If you dream you're back at school taking your exams for
example (one I'll cover later), it might be you wake up singing a
song you associate with that time in your life.

If you wake up singing a song you haven't heard in a while,
you could pause to see if there is a part of your history it's from
that is relevant to your life now. As you'll see in my thoughts
about how to work with dreams, key questions to reflect on and
why this (e.g. song) and why now?

4) Lyrics as Information. In the years before we wrote stuff down, we passed on wisdom to our tribe through songs and storytelling. For example, in Buddhist tradition the teachings of Shakyamuni Buddha are believed to have been handed down through chanting, for around 400 years.

It's possible that the lyrics of the song you've woken up with provide some insight or information that could be useful, so it's worth writing the lyrics down and seeing how you interpret them.

If you find you have this experience regularly, keeping a dream diary might help. You can see if there are any patterns as to why you wake up with those lyrics and their possible meaning. (A Dream Record Example is at the back.)

Keep in mind, there could be lots of reasons this is happening which are still unexplored – the song might reflect your mood, a memory or just be a song.

5) Inspiration. Several people throughout history have woken up with a tune on their lips and used this as the inspiration for their own music creations.

Keith Richards reportedly dreamt the riff for *(I Can't Get No) Satisfaction* just as Paul McCartney apparently dreamt the tune for *Yesterday*. So if you don't recognise the song you're humming when you wake up, maybe write it down or record it. (I heard that Keith Richards kept a guitar and tape player by his bed just in case.) Who knows, we may be hearing your song in the charts very soon!

One thing Williamson's research did highlight is how different we all are. In a database of "ear worms" of over 2500 songs, it was rare that people had the same "stuck song".

Just like our dreams and their meanings are unique to each of us, this highlights our individuality and the way we interpret the music we hear.

Hopefully, what I've written so far is starting to reassure you that the dark can bring some answers, or at least might not be as scary now as you were once taught to believe. A lot of what we feel at night is normal and manageable, and can in fact provide useful insights in what positive steps we take next. Let's explore now what you could try when you can't sleep.

## Safe Enough to Sleep

*Though sleep is called our best friend, it is a friend who often keeps us waiting!*
~ Jules Verne

If you're someone who hasn't been sleeping well for a while, you'll know that sinking feeling when you realise you are wide awake in bed, and everyone else is asleep.

Whilst I explained earlier this may be because of an instinctive "sentinel" reflex to stay alert and care for your family (albeit on a subconscious level), it won't necessarily change the fact that you're now laying in bed staring at the ceiling, or help you get back to sleep. It's the same if you live on your own; it's generally accepted that your brain's number one priority is survival, so it makes sense if you find yourself awake, looking out for yourself. (This isn't selfish, it's instinctive.)

The key to addressing this may be to make sure you feel safe at night, so that's what we'll explore next. Feeling safe could also improve your dream content, or reduce experiences like the "Old Hag Syndrome" and "First Night Effect" I described earlier. We'll then look a bit more at how to manage the mind – and your grief – if you've identified that's what's stopping you.

Safety in sleep can start with your bedtime routine, which is one reason I promote something called "The Golden Hour" or the One Hour Rule, the 60 minutes (or so) before bedtime when you set yourself up for a good night sleep.

## The Golden Hour/The One Hour Rule

According to the Royal Society for Public Health, sleep is as vital for survival as food and water.[62]

I touched lightly earlier on some of the side effects of not getting enough sleep, but you'll know yourself how this affects you, especially if you're recognising some early warning signs. You might have already decided to put sleep higher up your to-do list, but don't really know where to start. Setting the intention each day to make room for sleep can make the process easier in itself.

If you've been considering some of the ideas in this book already, you might have started to notice a pattern developing around your sleep cycle, for example when you feel naturally sleepy at night or when you wake up as the sun rises in the morning.

You might have identified that historically you've been someone who tends to "push through" sleepiness, which means you then can't sleep when you eventually head up to bed; again this is why winding down can be so helpful.

The Golden Hour for sleep essentially recognises that what you do in the space before bedtime can make the difference to a good night's sleep or not. (Incidentally, in policing the "Golden Hour" means something completely different; this is definitely not that.)

If you're someone who checks social media late in to the evening (I think we are all guilty of that), answers work emails or generally does anything which could potentially disrupt your body clock (like eating a heavy meal or exercising late at night), you might not sleep so well.

Even if you feel naturally sleepy and go to bed then, it can still help to begin the process of winding down an hour before. As an example, if you feel naturally sleepy around 10pm, it would mean that by 9pm you've finished any chores and written your "to-do" list for the next day. If you're not sure yet when you feel naturally sleepy, you could set what you think would be a reasonable bedtime, and then try the Golden Hour and see if it helps, adjusting over time based on how easy/hard it feels to fall asleep.

When you were younger, and if you were lucky enough, your parents or caregivers may have given you a bath, a warm milky drink and a bedtime story. It seems just as important as we get older, it's just that we think we should have grown out of it.

You could also put on some calming music in the background and see if that helps; I mentioned the *Goldberg Aria* earlier, and I'm sure Classic FM have a kind of "Bedtime Hour" (Smooth Classics) for this very reason. Another thing to try is mindfulness which I'll explore a lot more in a section later on.

## Night Time Checklist

If it helps with feeling physically safe, you may also decide to establish an additional routine, of going round checking doors, windows and appliances, and, if you have one, setting a house alarm. You can literally create a check list if it feels helpful, as long as it doesn't become a chore or a problem in itself that gets in the way of a good night's sleep (e.g. if it has the potential to become an *amplifier*, like I've described earlier).

When I've worked with victims of crime, they've found having outside security lights helpful where possible, both to act as reassurance and as a deterrent, alongside making sure your phone is fully charged or nearby, or getting hold of a panic alarm if needed.

You may find you have a "Bobby Scheme" through your local police service who can help with a safety check of your premises, and may even be able to signpost you to some free or reasonably priced local services that can help you feel more secure in your home. If you live in social/affordable accommodation, your housing association should also be able to help.

If you have been a victim of crime and this is one of the reasons you struggle to sleep at night, then there are services set up to help you (a list of useful links is at the back of the book), who can also make referrals as needed.

If you decide to go through a series of safety checks before you go to bed, try to do this *before* the Golden Hour, so that you're not using up your sleepiness worrying about locking up. You can always do a final quick check as you're heading to bed if you feel it's helpful.

Sometimes though, what compromises our feelings of safety can actually be the boundaries we have (or not) in place at home. If you can, it's good to let friends and family know for example that you won't check your phone after a certain time of night.

Before mobile phones, it was never socially acceptable to ring after a certain time in the evening, or before a certain time in the morning, and just because we're technically available now 24/7 via technology, doesn't mean we have to be literally. Don't be afraid to have a voicemail which says if people ring you after 9pm (for example) you won't be calling them back until the next day. If you have a smartphone you can set up "favourites" so that only certain people can get through when your phone is on Do Not Disturb.

## Bedroom Environment

Where you sleep is a key player in helping you get a decent night's rest. We know that room temperature is important, because your body needs it cool to help with the process of falling asleep. When a room is too hot, you're more likely to feel uncomfortable (this may in itself cause nightmares) so it makes sense that you'll struggle to stay asleep too.

Just as your dog or cat may have a preferred place to sleep at night, humans are not much different. This is one of the reasons we suffer with the First Night Effect I mentioned earlier, because our brain feels safer in a bed that we know and love. You might also find blackout curtains helpful to keep out the light, especially if you live in a well-lit area. Here are some things to think about:

## A Sleep Sanctuary – Key Ingredients

Is your bedroom cluttered, or is there space to move around? A "busy" environment may lead to feelings of discomfort, so try to keep your bedroom clear and tidy.

What are the colours like in your room? "Warm colours" including orange, red and yellows can help your environment feel more soothing, and lend itself to rest.

What temperature is your room? The optimum room temperature is thought to be around 16-18 degrees Celsius or 60-65 degrees Fahrenheit. (Young children and older people may need the room a little warmer so keeping a thermometer in the room can help.) Anything over 24 degrees Celsius (71 degrees Fahrenheit) might make you restless[63] and you'll find it harder to drop off. As I've said, a room that's too hot may also contribute to nightmares, which can be one reason you wake up sweating (another might be stress).

Is your bedding suitable? Cotton sheets are generally recommended as you're less likely to get too sweaty at night. If you can afford it, use blankets as an extra layer in winter, and change your duvet in the summer months (or just use the duvet cover when it gets really warm). Don't necessarily buy in to the hype about how often you should change your mattress, some manufacturers say eight years, where others say 15. The main thing is if it's comfortable and clean, it's probably doing its job.

Do you keep your phone by your bed? I've mentioned how it can help you feel safe, but where you can, leave it in another room and if possible use an alarm clock that doesn't glare (or frighten the life out of you when it wakes you up).

Are there sounds that keep you awake? It's not always possible to block out background noise – the activities in the pages on mindfulness might help.

Lighting: Warm colours can have a soporific effect, so instead of having a 100w bulb in your overhead light, you might invest in one with a softer glow for your nightstand if you have one.

*Nod to Colour: Whereas your brain may process the "blue" light from your phone as daylight, it doesn't seem to mind soft yellows or oranges, like the type you'd find in a lit fireplace. If you've ever found yourself dozing off in front of a cosy fire in winter, that might well be why.*

*This could mean a soothing "warm" glow from a night light could help with sleepiness, and be less likely to keep you awake. If you do need an alarm clock, try not to use your phone but one that takes these warm colours in to account. Smartphone manufacturers may try to persuade you their filters manage the "blue light", but if your mind is active from scrolling on your device, you're not going to head for the land of nod.*

## What Else Can Help You Sleep

There are a lot of different remedies and solutions you can try, as I said earlier sleep aids are big business. You can try an eye mask, ear plugs, lavender bubble bath, a foot rub, even scented creams and candles all designed to help you relax (never leave a candle lit when you're trying to nod off, obviously).

My main word of caution about these, is that if you rely on them too heavily, they in themselves become a problem. (I mentioned earlier, Dr Guy Meadows refers to these as *amplifiers*.) Try not to over-rely on sleep solutions, and instead just consider them as a treat in your bedtime routine that you can take or leave. If you start saying things like "I *need* my scented eye mask to help me sleep!", you might start stressing, your mind start spiralling and that's not conducive to rest at all.

Some people suggest that there is an optimum position for sleep, but again just find what works for you.

If it's worries about the week ahead, or thoughts that pop in to your head, keep a pen and paper by the bed so you can write them down when you need, to deal with them later, and give yourself permission to let them wait until tomorrow. Having a journal by your bed can also help you record your dreams if you have them; more on that soon.

Mindfulness is another proven strategy for healthy sleep and I've included a load of activities on this further on.

### Activity – Tracking Your Sleep

I mentioned earlier that some people track their sleep through their fit bit, but this in itself has created a new anxiety called Orthosomnia. For that reason, it might be more helpful to resort to good old pen and paper.

The table below offers a template to design your own sleep record in your notebook. This could help monitor how many times you're waking and possible reasons, so that if you need to you can discuss this with your doctor.

| Date | Time to Bed | No. Times Waking | Reason for Waking | How Long Awake | What Helped You Fall Back to Sleep |
|------|-------------|------------------|-------------------|----------------|-----------------------------------|
|      |             |                  |                   |                |                                   |
|      |             |                  |                   |                |                                   |
|      |             |                  |                   |                |                                   |
|      |             |                  |                   |                |                                   |

I mentioned earlier that researchers used to suggest (and some still do) that if you find yourself awake in the night, and don't nod back off within 20 minutes, to get up and go back to bed when you're sleepy.

I tend not to advise this anymore because the brain can adapt to that as a new habit or routine; the next time you wake up your brain seems to assume getting up is just what you now do.

If you resonated with my bus analogy, you might find you're feeling sleepy if Sleep Pressure rebuilds again anyway, whether you get up or not, so staying in bed at least means you can rest. If you feel you have to get up (i.e. because you need the toilet) or you are getting more stressed just laying in bed, then do get up. Just make sure you do something boring, that won't stimulate you. If, however, you feel you can stay in bed at least to rest, even if you can't sleep, then the activity that follows might help.

## *Activity for Middle of the Night Waking*

1. Acknowledge you're awake. Try not to think about why, or what for. Simply acknowledge that's where you are right now. If it's because you've forgotten to do something, you could just say "Thank you" to your mind and make a note, either in your mind or with the pen and paper you have by the bed.

2. Be kind to yourself. Whatever the reason you've woken up, try to avoid punishing or reprimanding yourself – your brain won't help you sleep if you're beating yourself up. You could repeat a mantra in your mind that helps you feel relaxed, something like: "Right now, it's like this," or "It is what it is."

3. Breathe. If you find it helpful, bring your awareness gently to your breath. Notice where it's coming in and going out of your body. You might notice you're breathing in your nose, or out through your mouth. There is no right or wrong way to breathe, your body knows how much air you need. Simply notice that you're breathing, and where the breath finds its way in and out of your body. If you find paying attention to your breath difficult, just rest your hand on your tummy and notice how the tummy rises and falls as you breathe. As you breathe, you could

try another mantra like, "Breathing in, I calm my body; breathing out, I calm my mind."

# The Mind and Sleep

*The mind can be a beautiful servant, and a dangerous master.*
~ Unknown

The mind is a powerful thing. Much like sleep, it can be our friend, or feel like the enemy. When it's working well, we progress, we work, we're creative and we flourish. When it's not, it can feel like the darkness creeps inside.

I've explored already how the dark can make things feel more intense, and in the wake of a global crisis, everything seems magnified. Whilst in the personal story I described earlier the initial answer for me came from someone else, moments of deep and helpful reflection can arrive in the quiet of night. Where dreams can echo fears and our pain, they can also offer motivation and hope.

When I found myself desperate in the dark all those years ago, it was largely because of the way I was talking to myself.

And I know I'm not alone.

Research supports that what keeps so many of us awake at night is not just our situation, but what we think about it. Even thinking we're not going to get enough sleep, ironically, can get in the way of us nodding off. Whatever our circumstances, how we interpret what's happening – i.e. what does this mean *for* me or *about* me – can trigger fight or flight, and well, the notion of sleep will make a sharp exit.

Researchers like Jill Bolte Taylor have discovered that when we feel a strong emotion, it takes just 90 seconds to run its course in the body.[64] What keeps it going, is the meaning we attach to it and how we think.

If we had an argument with a friend earlier in the day, it's not the row that's keeping us up; it's done, it's not in the here and now. What's stopping us sleeping is the thoughts about what we should (or shouldn't) have said, or what we should have done. Even physical pain, or something natural like the menopause, can keep us more awake at night if we're asking ourselves, "Why me?" or "Why now?"

However you're feeling right now, it's valid. I hope you've been able to capture from this book already that whether you identify with grief, and the impact it can have or not, your emotions matter just like you do. So when you find yourself awake at night, it's worth learning how to manage the mind.

Ask someone who says they can't sleep what they've tried and they'll say "everything"; ask someone who sleeps well what they do to achieve it, they'll reply "nothing".

This is where mindfulness can help.

## Mind Management

The concept of mindfulness is over 2500 years old, and originated in the time of Shakyamuni, the historical Buddha, who was born Siddhārtha Gautama. Mindfulness is not a religion, more an intelligent philosophy which focuses on easing the mental anguish we know today as stress, anxiety and depression.

The Buddha recognised that inevitably we all – every human – want just two things: to avoid pain, and to be happy (I don't know anyone who wakes up in the morning and says, "I hope I have a miserable day today"). Our shared unity in these two common goals is what is known as our "common humanity".

The problem is that striving for those very things can create problems of their own, what the Buddha referred to as the cause of suffering. We pursue happiness by seeking perfection, and we seek to avoid pain by distracting and numbing out.

Mindfulness gives us the opportunity to recognise what we're thinking and how we're feeling, but without getting caught up in the commentary about what caused it. It's the "what", not the "why". So if you notice you often have thoughts about "what if" and "if only", mindfulness can help you manage the feelings our thoughts create.

Mindfulness is giving your focused awareness to the present moment, without judgement. It's an ethical system of investigation that enables you to listen to your body, and manage (even tame) the mind in such a way that rather than your mind driving you to distraction, you can take the wheel.

You've probably been mindful more times than you realise. If you've ever caught yourself listening to the birds singing, or the rain on your windowsill during a storm, then you've already been practising.

Whether you're walking, sitting in a meeting or having a cup of tea, you can use the experience of what you're doing in that moment to keep you right where you are. It's immersing yourself and leaning in to whatever is happening, but without judging how it should or shouldn't be. You'd probably never look at a beautiful sunset, and say, "It's okay but it needs a bit more orange in the top left"; you'd accept it just as it is. That's what I mean when I say mindfulness acknowledges the what of the present moment, without getting caught up in the why.

In Western society, we often find it hard to show self-compassion or make room for ourselves. You might feel lazy or guilty if you stop to unwind. You might beat yourself up if you make a mistake, or when you feel you're not measuring up in some area of your life. Perhaps you lash out at people, or hide yourself away when you're going through a difficult time. But these are just habits. We weren't born judging ourselves or behaving like this, they are patterns that have developed over time, potentially because we believed they help us feel safe.

Mindfulness includes learning about kindness, compassion and non-judgement towards yourself. Instead of pushing experiences away and then reacting out of habit, mindfulness invites you to notice what's happening, so that you can learn to control how you behave when things are difficult.

With the exciting discovery of neuroplasticity – the knowledge that we can change – we know now that with time and effort, we can change direction; practice makes peaceful. Instead of our brain reacting in the same way as it's always done, we can teach it to behave in a new and healthier way. We can become the observer of our thoughts, rather than the participant.

When we feel stressed or under pressure, our immune system can be impacted; it's one reason we get sick the minute we take some leave. This is why rest and relaxation are so important, especially for busy people; Mindfulness can be a useful – and not-too-time-consuming – approach to coping.

## Mindfulness and Meditation

I make an important distinction that mindfulness and meditation are not the same. Mindfulness is about being aware, and you can do that anywhere: at home, at work, on the bus, in the doctor's surgery, even in the dentist's chair. Meditation is a more formal practice of resting in one of the postures with the intention to be mindful. It's not about posing cross-legged on the floor with your hands in mudra (although to be fair, you can if you want to). The key point is, the more you do, the better you become.

## Ways to be Mindful without Meditating

Not everyone finds they can sit still for a meditation practice, at least not straight away and not with their eyes closed. If you've suffered a trauma meditation is not always recommended, in case the stillness brings up uncomfortable thoughts or sensations.

Most of us will find, especially in the early days, that being left alone with our thoughts for too long can be challenging; this is why our thoughts cause so many problems at night.

Having a teacher can help, especially one who approaches mindfulness and meditation with a trauma-informed approach. But there are ways you can be mindful without sitting with your eyes closed. You can:

- do some mindful colouring
- sing your heart out to your favourite song
- repeat a word, phrase or mantra like the ones I mentioned earlier: "It is what it is" or "Right now, it's like this" (I'll offer more later)
- go for a walk and pay attention to all the colours you can see
- sit and drink a cup of tea, and appreciate the connection to all the people who helped you make it (the people who picked and packed the tea, provided the electricity in to your home, the person in the supermarket who put it on the shelves, and so on)
- doing the washing up, feeling the warmth of the water and suds on your hands as you clean each item in the bowl.

## What mindfulness is not:

x – clearing the mind: This is one of the biggest misconceptions of mindfulness. In fact, when researchers have asked people to try and clear their mind – even those who described themselves as happy, with no money worries, no work problems and no relationship difficulties (I don't know where they found them) – the longest they could manage is about seven seconds; that was pre-COVID. The mind is designed to think, that's its job. So trying to empty the mind is unnatural, and actually pretty boring too. Your mind just wants something to do, mindfulness gives it a job.

With mindfulness we can *manage* the mind. So as the mind wanders off, which it inevitably does, we just notice that and bring it back to what we're trying to pay attention to. Think of it like training a puppy, every time it chases off, we ask it to come back and "stay".

x – "new age woo-woo": I've mentioned already that mindfulness is around 2500 years old. It's not new age, even though many people think it arrived in the 60s on the back of the Beatles. It's been around a long time, and for that reason suggests there may well be something good in it.

x – a clinical strategy: Mindfulness is not really a tool, or a solution as such, it's more a way of life. Whilst some people may think it's a panacea for healing, the reality is it's not for everyone.

Trying to be mindful towards your body, for example, won't work if you hate the way you look, and actually that can be quite distressing. This is why I suggest people speak to their healthcare team first, and discuss whether or not now is the right time for you.

As you get more used to being mindful, you'll find you do it more and more in everything you do. It has no specific purpose, but has many benefits.

## What are the benefits?

The research on mindfulness and meditation is growing every year. In their book *The Science of Meditation*, Daniel Goleman and Richard J. Davidson say:

> *In the 1970's, when we began publishing our research on meditation, there were a just handful of scientific articles on the topic. At last count there numbered 6,838 such articles, with a notable acceleration of late. For 2014, the annual number was 925... in 2016, there were 1,113 such publications in the English language scientific literature.*

The benefits include being a proven technique for:

- Effective relaxation
- Reducing stress and improving mental health
- Managing pain
- Improving the immune system

- Enhanced concentration
- Lowering blood pressure
- Better sleep and reducing insomnia

## How long should I try this for?

Whether you're trying seated meditation or just spending time being mindful in nature, you can practise for 90 seconds each day (including when you feel emotions rising) or you can take longer if you have the time. The more you practise, the sooner you'll see results.

## The Mind Needs a Home

My mindfulness teacher is a very modern monk, so trendy in fact that his mobile phone matches his robes. He prefers lemon and ginger tea, and loves rose-scented incense. He usually starts every conversation with a joke but most importantly taught me a fair majority of what I now teach in mindfulness – that was part of the "deal" as he put it; he teaches me what he knows, and I pass it on. He has been my teacher for many years, and always will be (when you sign up for a life of service in this way, that's just how these things work).

One of the most profound things he ever said to me, is that the mind needs a home. Anything that is homeless, is usually unhappy. This is why we need to help the mind find its way back.

Mindfulness is the opposite of being on automatic pilot. Where you might reactively behave in one way when you're upset, the mind has become homeless. When you're mindful you consciously choose what you're doing next to bring the mind back home.

When they can't sleep at night, people tell me it's usually because of their thoughts. Not always worry, but nevertheless the constant whirring of a noisy mind. Being able to control the mind is key to getting a good night's sleep, even when you're going through a difficult time.

The activities I will describe next can help you notice unhelpful thinking before it becomes a problem, or challenge it helpfully if it does, even if it's the middle of the night. The most common reason people tell me they give up on mindfulness and meditation is because they think they're doing it wrong. Hopefully, as you'll see, it's easier than you might think.

## When Not to Practise

Mindfulness and Meditation have been proven to help people feel calm, and especially helpful to manage mild to moderate stress, depression and anxiety, and in many ways grief.

There may be times when meditation feels like the last thing on your mind. This is when applying a mindfulness activity – like noticing the rain on your windowsill or your hand on your belly – can be a more helpful way to manage the mind.

If you have suffered a trauma though, or have a severe and enduring mental health consideration you may wish to speak to your healthcare team before trying the following activities. You may also wish to speak with them if you suffer with asthma or heart conditions, or have any concerns particularly for the activities that focus on the breath or the body. Do what's healthy and feels right for you.

## Mindfulness Activities for Bedtime (and Beyond)

Another common myth about mindfulness and meditation is that you can't do it in bed. I absolutely disagree with this, and when I've taught people these techniques for night-time they've found them really helpful. In the original teachings, one of the postures for meditation is laying down, so you're not breaking any rules if you are being mindful or meditate this way.

Whilst falling asleep isn't usually the goal of mindful meditation (if it had one, it would be managing the mind), it's a happy side effect if you drift off in to a lovely refreshing sleep.

Start with one activity and see how you get on, trying it for a few minutes or longer if it helps. Work your way through the activities at your own pace, maybe trying a different one each night. If you find one more helpful than another, stick with that for a while.

## Mindfulness Activities for Sleep

1. When you're in bed, bring your awareness to the experience of laying down only. Start at your feet, and just notice how they're feeling right now, and how your toes feel next to each other. Then pay attention to how your back feels resting where it is, and then your hands resting on the duvet. It might feel warm or cold, soft or smooth. If your mind starts to wander, that's okay – that's what busy minds do. Every time you notice your mind has wandered off, just acknowledge that and try not to beat yourself up. Bring your awareness once again to the experience of laying down. If it's helpful repeat the words "laying down" in your mind, because that's what you're doing. Try this for a few minutes if it helps. An extension of this activity is to try a body scan. I've offered a more detailed script further on.

2. When we are stressed our breath is one of the first things affected; our breathing can become shallow which in itself can lead to headaches, and more feelings of stress. It's not that we need to think about breathing all the time (thankfully your body does that naturally, giving you one less thing to worry about) but it can be helpful to notice the breath and bring your conscious awareness to it. Laying down, with one hand on your belly and one on your chest, simply notice their movement as you breathe in and out. Just sink into the natural rhythm of your breathing, without judgement or worrying if it's too fast or slow. Your body knows how much air you need.

3. Similar to the activity above, you can try an exercise in self-compassion by literally placing your hand over your heart. This activity can soothe tension and help you relax. Simply place

your hand on your chest, over the heart area, and bring your awareness to how it feels to be showing yourself kindness this way. If you want to, take three slow, deep breaths if you can. You can also add a mantra like, "May I show myself kindness and find peace in this moment."

4. S.T.O.P.P. is an acronym that can be applied in many settings, especially when dealing with difficult emotions.[65] The S stands for stop, in that you can literally ask yourself to stop what you're doing. Sometimes, when feelings are overwhelming, just saying the word "stop" to yourself (or out loud) can be enough to interrupt your thoughts. The T is for Take a Breath, so similar to the activities earlier, just notice that you're breathing. O stands for observing, so that you can notice what's going on in your body right now as you feel the way you do. Again, you're not judging this, you're just labelling it as it is. Instead of describing tension in your body for example, you could label it as sensation. If it helps, place your hand on where the tension is and say in your mind, "Here it is." Remember you're not focusing on why it's there or what or who caused it, you're just acknowledging where it is, because it's there anyway. The first P is for Perspective, where you might allow yourself for a moment to consider that there is a wider picture than what we can see. You don't have to think about what that might be just yet, just acknowledge there probably is one. For example, you might acknowledge that you don't know that you won't sleep, only what you've told yourself. Then the last P is for Proceed, with help. It might be that you're relaxed enough to sleep, but that you resolve to ask for help if you need it.

5. It's easy to get hooked by our thinking, and to believe what our mind is telling us. But our thoughts are only a problem if we believe them; thoughts about worry are not facts, *especially* not at 4am. One thing you can try every time you notice that your mind is wandering is literally just describe in your mind what you're doing, which is thinking. Repeat the word "thinking" in

your mind every time you realise it's happening, then return your attention to where you are now, or focusing on your breath. You don't need to tell yourself off for thinking, remember your brain is just doing its job. Instead, just set the intention to focus on the here and now, notice your mind wanders, describe what you're doing, then go back to your intention to be here now. Notice. Label. Return. Repeat.

6. Begin by making yourself comfortable in bed and give yourself permission to relax. Take three deep breaths, and as you exhale extend the breath a little, and allow tension to leave your body; feel yourself become more and more relaxed as you breathe out. Return your breathing to its natural steady rhythm, then if you want to, imagine that you are in a safe space perhaps on a well-deserved holiday. It might be somewhere you know, or it could be completely imaginary. It could be a secret walled garden or a luxury palace that is yours to design. Notice everything about this place, including the sights and sounds, and the peace it brings. You can imagine yourself surrounded by a warm protective light with a vibrant glow, or protective cloak or shield if this helps you feel safe. Everything about this place is warm, comforting and sacred, and only you have the key or the map to visit. Imagine what you'd be doing in this peaceful place: you might be enjoying a sunrise, or watching the waves roll in to shore. If you don't fall asleep, when you're ready, leave this special place in your imagination, keeping with you the feelings of warmth and relaxation, and know that you can return in your mind when you need to feel calm and at peace.

7. Mantras are a word or phrase you can repeat in your mind, for as long as it's helpful, to keep your attention in one place. I've mentioned a couple already, but here are some more you can adapt or try. Sometimes we won't always feel able to use a positive "I" statement like "I am happy", so you can change the sentence structure to turn this in to an aspiration, for example

"May I be happy". You can repeat these in your mind as many times as feel helpful, and could use them alongside any of the activities above.

1.  I give myself permission to rest.
2.  I deserve to relax.
3.  May I wake up refreshed, with feelings of purpose and joy.
4.  As everything changes, may I remain at ease.[66]
5.  All is well in my life (or May all be well in my life).
6.  May I be happy, loving myself right here, right now.
7.  I accept myself. I belong here.
8.  I allow harmony in to my life.
9.  May I experience what life offers with kindness.
10. I am learning to be kind to myself.

## Full Body Scan Meditation

When I've taught this next activity in my classes, most people come back the following week and say they didn't get above the knees before they fell asleep. However, because a body scan is bringing your awareness to your body, it's important to consider if this is the right one for you. If you don't mind focusing on how your body feels, then this is how to start.

Just as in the activity above, where you focused on laying down, start in the same way. Bring your awareness to the experience of being in bed, and noticing how it feels to be resting where you are. Give yourself permission to relax, and if your mind wanders at any time, just notice that and return your attention to the activity, without judging. If you find yourself distracted by sounds like a car going by or a door slamming outside, just label them for what they are – which is "sound" – and again return to the activity. There are no right or wrong sounds, so they can become part of this activity. It might feel strange paying attention to sounds if they're annoying, but by giving them your full attention, you might find they become less distracting.

Turn your attention towards your feet and notice how they feel to be resting where they are right now. Slowly bring your awareness around to your ankles, your heels and then to the tops of your feet. Notice how your toes feel, resting next to each other. If you notice any tension stored in these places, label it in your mind as "sensation" then take a deep breath as if you're breathing in to those places, and then feel the tension ease as you exhale, returning to a natural steady rhythm. Continue slowly up your shins, around to your calves and in to your knees. Again notice if any tension is stored in these places, label it as "sensation" then take a deep breath as if you're breathing in relaxation to where you feel the tension is stored. Return your breathing to a natural steady rhythm. Continue up your body, doing this with different parts of your body, including if you want to, your thighs, pelvis, buttocks, tummy, chest, arms, hands, elbows, neck, shoulders, back of the head, top of the head, forehead and face. Finally bring your attention in to your back if you want to, remembering to notice, breathe and release each time, returning the breath to a natural steady rhythm. If you haven't fallen asleep, you can just bring your attention once again to your breath or the experience of laying down for as long as you find that helpful.

If you want to make this activity longer, instead of coming up the body from both feet for example, you could start by coming up the right side of your body and return down the left, and extending even more by coming up the left side of your body and going down the right.

Remember you don't have to get up in the night to help you sleep better, so if it's more helpful to stay in bed so that at least your body can rest even if you can't sleep, the body scan may help.

## A Guided Meditation for Difficult Times

COVID-19 has affected us all in different ways, and there isn't a single person on the planet who hasn't been touched by it in some way especially through grief and loss.

When we are sad or anxious, we can isolate and withdraw. We can feel like no one else in the world understands how we feel. But the common humanity I described earlier means, even when we feel lonely, we are not alone. Somewhere in the world right now, someone understands because they are feeling it too.

When you feel frightened, or worried, when you feel annoyed or even numb, in a planet of nearly 8 billion people, there is someone who feels as you do right now.

It might not be for the same reasons; your problems right now may be completely unique to you. But even so, there will be someone somewhere feeling anger, sadness, worry and more.

Mindfulness gives you permission to experience the present moment just as it is even when it's difficult, but without getting caught up in the commentary about why it is like it is. We call this leaning in or sitting with the difficult. Pushing pain away rarely helps in the long run, because we don't really push it away. Remember, the etymology of the word "depressed" means something that's been pushed down, just as anger can be unexpressed fear or grief. If we keep pretending pain isn't there, inevitably it will rise up in ways that can be unhelpful.

So mindfulness is being where you are right now, just as it is, without getting caught up in unhealthy thinking, or hooked by how things – or people – should be. Mindfulness helps us to recognise what we can and can't control; that we can learn to pick our battles, or at least what we choose to think about.

We know that the breath is one way to help relax the mind and body; it can be a switch between the subconscious and the conscious mind. It can activate the relaxation response, and calm fight or flight. It can take you from a place of "I can't cope" to "I can cope".

A loving kindness meditation is an acknowledgement of common humanity. It allows you to connect with others who may be feeling as you do, when you're going through a difficult time, and is an act of compassion – of giving and receiving – both towards yourself and others. Where it can feel selfish to indulge in an act of self-care, this style of meditation can reassure you that whilst you take a moment for yourself, you are offering a gesture of kindness towards others too.

Here is an example:

- Make yourself as comfortable as possible, and gently bring your awareness to the experience of sitting or laying down where you are. Your mind will wander, and that's okay. Every time your mind goes off, notice that, describe it in your mind without judgement simply as "thinking" (because that's what you're doing) and then return your attention to sitting or laying down, repeating "sitting" or "laying down" as many times as you need, to keep your mind in one place.
- Gently turn your attention to your breath and just notice that you're breathing. We don't need to worry about what that looks like or why, just sink in to the natural rhythm of your breath knowing it has the capacity to relax your body and mind.
- As you breathe in, acknowledge that this breath is for you, as it helps activate a relaxation response to calm your body and mind. If you want, and if it's helpful, you can say in your mind, "I breathe in for me."
- As you breathe out, keep the people in your mind who may be feeling as you do right now, whether they're known or unknown, as an act of compassionate solidarity with them whoever they may be. If you want, and if it's helpful, you can say in your mind, "I breathe out for you," wherever they are in the world right now. Remember these don't have to be deep breaths, just natural as they come.

You can do this activity anywhere it feels safe to do so, whether in the supermarket, sat at your desk or laying in bed.

Some of the activities described here will be available to access free of charge for people who have bought this book in the resources section of the website when this book is published at https://answersinthedark.com/resources (password sleepwell). There are other apps you may have already tried to practise mindfulness, with a focus on sleep, like Headspace and Calm. The only thing to keep in mind with third-party apps, is that some of the features may be behind a paywall.

# Part III

# Put Your Dreams to Bed

*Faith sees best in the dark.*

~ Søren Kierkegaard

Dreams have been described as the window in to our soul. They speak to us in ways that can be useful, but can also cause fear and panic, at least when they're misunderstood.

Some people may dread going to sleep in case they have a bad dream and, ironically, the more stressed we are, the more frightening our dream content might be. But dreams are good for you, and this section aims to explain why we don't have to be afraid of them.

Their wisdom can be as helpful as that of a good friend. In fact, Swansea University Sleep Laboratory found that discussing a dream for approximately an hour can result in "a-ha" moments for people:

> *These can include realisations of where items of dream content came from in waking life, and of metaphorical references to particular concerns, issues or events – that may not have been easily seen or understood during waking hours.*

They also suggest that sharing our dreams can even help improve relationships.[67]

This is how dreams can help you heal.

For a long time dreams have been misrepresented or ignored; in our busy modern world, we might even ask what relevance they have at all. I've seen prominent speakers in the world of sleep science tell us to ignore them (which understandably sends dream researchers, who have made it their life's work, in to a bit of a spin). Others boil them down to a random set of images that we have in our minds at night. If that were true, we wouldn't be able to make sense of our dreams, at least not the ones that happen in REM sleep.

The value of dreams has been proven, time and again. And ultimately, we can't stop them happening, so we might as well explore how we can make them work to our advantage.

The changes we've seen in our sleep and dreaming habits since COVID-19 have highlighted that there's more going on in our minds, than what we scratch the surface with every day.

In the pages that follow, I will be sharing what I've learned in a lifetime so far of helping people, which offers food for thought, alongside tips that might help. This isn't a prescription of what dreams mean, nor is it a dream dictionary, but an honest look at what they are, how they can help and where to start in understanding them.

Our fear of dreams is nothing new. For hundreds of years, exploring dreams was seen as messing with unknown forces, in some cases people did (and still do) conflate dream interpretation with devil worship. People are so scared their dreams make them look weird, or that something is wrong with them – which has rarely, if ever, been the case in my experience – they're too scared to speak of them.

## What Are Dreams?

The stage most associated with dreaming is Rapid Eye Movement or REM sleep, and it's thought to be associated most with learning and remembering. At the beginning of the night you're dreaming for roughly five to 10 minutes, and by the time you wake up, you could have had a dream which lasted three-quarters of an hour (or more). But what are they?

At the very front of this book I included the Oxford English Dictionary definition of dreams which says:

*1. a series of thoughts, images, and sensations occurring in a person's mind during sleep.*

What I love about this description is that it acknowledges that we experience dreams in many ways, not just in images. Blind people dream, and they tell me, if blind since birth, it's like listening to the radio. Others who have lost their sight over time said they love their sleep, because they can see again in their dreams.

You can taste in a dream, just as you can smell and touch. People describe experiences of enjoying a tasty sandwich, or drinking a glass of water and wake up to find they were hungry or thirsty. Others notice the smell of a flower, or the touch of a thorn. In none of these cases, did the dreamer awake to find the sign of crumbs or a rose in their bed; their experiences were exclusive to that period of REM sleep.

In the same way, if we are laying funny in bed at night, and we wake with pins and needles in our hand, we might have dreamt the thorn has pricked us in the fingers. The pressure or pain we experience, whilst asleep, can manifest in our dreams, something known as "somatic phenomena". In *The Nightmare Encyclopedia*, Jeff Belanger and Kirsten Dalley write:

*The mind uses the dream to convey the uncomfortable state of our bodies, and because the dreaming mind doesn't present reality in the same way it does when we are awake, these messages often come to us in an exaggerated or symbolic way.*

You might notice that the definition of a dream says they occur "in a person's mind"; so it refers *not* to our brain, but in a space of possibility which isn't confined to grey matter itself. When scientists say they know about what part of our brain is responsible for dreaming, ultimately the mind isn't always where we think it is. This extract from an article explains:

*Where does the mind reside? It's a question that's occupied the best brains for thousands of years. Now, a patient who is self-aware –*

*despite lacking three regions of the brain thought to be essential for*
*self-awareness – demonstrates that the mind remains as elusive as*
*ever.*[68]

The way I describe them is that dreams are like a friend offering advice. Sometimes we pay attention. Sometimes we don't. But they create the possibility that we can connect what's in our awareness with what lays underneath, to bring about a sense of equilibrium. This is why I believe our dreams are so helpful if, for example, we have unresolved grief.

As David Fontana says in *Learn to Dream*:[69]

*Dreams are our chance to eavesdrop on a conversation between*
*our unconscious and conscious minds, offering us opportunities*
*to understand ourselves better and achieve greater inner harmony.*

Dreams can also be likened to a gift, one that only you can unwrap. Although dreams can be troubling, they are more like an encrypted, secret message with their own personal code. This means the dreamer already has everything they need to decide ultimately what they mean, even if they seem a mystery at first.

Although the subject has been talked about for thousands of years, and theorists have talked about their purpose, there is no fixed way to interpret them, or a special Enigma machine that can unravel their meaning. But this is a good thing. It means if you tell your neighbour the dream you had last night, whilst they might draw their own conclusions about what's going on in your life, they can never truly know. Ultimately, your privacy is protected within the sacred space of your mind.

This is why I always encourage people to explore dreams for themselves, with insights I will provide in this section. In the explanations I've offered about certain types of dreams in this book already, I've emphasised what they *could* mean, recognising that equally they might not.

If your dreams are really disturbing, it's okay to talk them through with someone who works in that field. It's still helpful that *you* create your personal library of definitions, based on your own exploration, rather than say rely on a dream dictionary which has only one point of view, and which most people say really gives nothing away.

Through my work I have been able to reassure hundreds, if not thousands, of people not only that there are things which can help achieve better sleep, but that the meanings of dreams are often less frightening than the dreams themselves; that once understood they seem to hold less power and certainly less fear over the person having them.

## Why do we dream?

Theory upon theory has been given about why we dream. Some people try to reduce this to the science of what part of our brain is responsible; others like myself look at the framework of the mind.

Many people recognise the name Sigmund Freud, just as they know Carl Jung, with others less well known like Alfred Adler or Jonathan Winson. Widely considered as "the founder of modern dream analysis", Winson formulated the theory that dreams evolved as a tool for remembering information important to survival and for consolidation of new and old memories.[70] And yet his is a name you might not have even heard.

Joe Griffin and Ivan Tyrrell have provided a new perspective of why we dream and what they mean, in their book *Dreaming Reality*. In Griffin's discovery of what he describes as the "expectation fulfilment theory of dreaming", the idea is that it's not our "emotionally arousing concerns" that influence our dreams, but our expectations not being met, or an opportunity not being presented to express ourselves in the way we wanted, during the day. This "unfinished business" then plays out in our dreams at night.

If you and I had a row for example, and I walk away thinking, "I should have said that," it may be my dream that night will present the opportunity to have my expectations met, and say my piece.

However, whilst all these theories are valid, in my experience, these aren't the only reasons we dream. Yes, what happens during the day can influence our dreams at night. But there's so much more than that.

If a researcher has a theory about why we dream, and uses their own dreams as the guiding principle, their dreams will confirm their theory because that's what they believe. (I know researchers obviously study more people, I'm just making the point that we can all potentially make research of dreams fit our theories, if we're using our own experiences as the concept; it's confirmation bias in action.) Our beliefs and backgrounds are some of the biggest factors which can influence what we dream and what they mean.

In the same way, if I only follow one way of working with dreams when I'm exploring them with someone, like believing Freud's principle that they're all just repressed desires, then I might only be looking at one side of the story.

In Rumi's *Masnavi*, he tells the story of the "Elephant in the Dark Room" (also known as "The Elephant and the Blind Men"), set in a city where all the inhabitants are reportedly blind. In the tale, a team of men are sent to examine an elephant, but each only had access to one part of the animal. Every one of the men believed, based on what part of the animal they were feeling, that they knew what it was, and what they were dealing with. Each perceived the animal from their own perspective. Interestingly, according to the story, each one of the men gained supporters, convinced that each description – and therefore each man – spoke the truth. This translation by EH Whinfield (1898) explains:[71]

*... as the place was too dark to permit them to see the elephant, they all felt it with their hands, to gain an idea of what it was like. One felt its trunk, and declared that the beast resembled a water-pipe; another felt its ear, and said it must be a large fan; another its leg, and thought it must be a pillar; another felt its back, and declared the beast must be like a great throne. According to the part which each felt, he gave a different description of the animal.*

I tell this story to highlight that because we're all so different, and whilst we can merit the relevance of all theories, we should keep an open mind.

When we work with dreams, it helps to remember that what might influence my dream content will be different to yours. If you look up the meaning of a dog in a dream dictionary, you'll perhaps see it symbolises a trusted and loyal friend. However, if you are afraid of dogs, your dream may mean something else. Our dreams can mean opposing things to each of us.

If one dream researcher says that your dreams are a projection of what happened the day before, that wouldn't explain why some people dream about a past life or a future event, sometimes with startling accuracy. (I'll come on to talk about this more.)

Carl Jung suggested that there may even be times where our dreams serve no other purpose than to bring us back to centre, without ever needing to understand their meaning. A visitation dream of a deceased loved one who appears fine and happy may be a perfect example of this; the dream itself might help us to move forward in our healing, with no other explanation needed. Ryan Hurd explains:

*Jung did not believe that dreams need to be interpreted for them to perform their function. Instead, he suggested that dreams are doing the work of integrating our conscious and unconscious lives; he called this the process of individuation.*[72]

Studies have also shown that as well as helping us make sense of our problems, the function of dreaming includes the storing of memory. In other words, it is having a dream tonight that will help you remember tomorrow what you did today. (If you haven't seen the Disney movie *Inside Out*, it explains this idea quite simply and brilliantly.)

*Nod to Dreaming Sleep: Mark Blagrove and his team at Swansea University have found that the emotional strength of what we experience during the day when we're awake can be linked to the content of our dreams. Their findings suggest that our most intense dreams occur when our brains are working hard to process recent, emotionally powerful experiences.*[73] *Dreams then are also a form of overnight therapy.*

## Why don't some people remember their dreams?
Like friends, if you ignore them long enough eventually dreams will leave you alone and you won't remember them anymore. Science tells us even if you don't remember your dreams you're still having them every night.

If you're not remembering them, there could be any number of reasons why.

For example:

- Our ability to remember our dreams will depend on the importance placed on them growing up. If you were always told your dreams don't mean anything as a child, you may well have subconsciously decided there's little value in remembering them.
- Women are more likely to remember their dreams than men.
- Smokers are less likely, and
- People who meditate are more likely than those who don't.[74]

172

People have told me they don't want to remember their dreams because they're scared of what they mean. One person told me they would deliberately try to stay awake all night if they thought a nightmare was likely.

I've mentioned, that lack of sleep ironically might increase your chance of nightmares, when you eventually doze off.

But as I hope I've been able to articulate throughout this book, we don't need to be afraid of the dark in ways we may have inherited previously, and we don't need to be scared of our dreams either – even the ones that startle us awake.

## Nightmares

Dreams are often symbolic messages to draw our attention to a specific situation. Sometimes the only time we might remember a dream is by the horrific nature of their content. We usually call this a nightmare.

In the book, *Nightmare*, Sandra Shulman writes:

*Since the beginning of recorded time the dream has occupied a prominent position in every culture and has exercised a profound effect, not only on the individual but also over religions and history. Dignified as a divine messenger, prophet, muse, problem-solver, route to the group unconscious, guardian of sleep, fulfiller of wishes, or signpost to psychological and physical ills, the dream has apparently opened a door into the unknown that could be of service to humanity. Its sister, the nightmare, enjoys equal significance, but for quite other reasons. Her unsolicited visits are so miserable that human beings have always wondered what purpose could be served by this grim invader of sleep.*[75]

Nightmares are "bad" dreams which can stay with us for hours, days or even years. They are often frightening, graphic and may cause you to wake up in a panic, crying or attempting to scream – that's really what separates them from other types of dreams.

Nightmares can be caused by a number of things. Lack of sleep, medication, bereavement, life-changing events, changes in diet and stress can all be a factor – even what you watch before you go to bed. As we've seen, just a room being too hot may be enough to cause a bad dream, which is why you wake up sweating, although the stress of the dream could have the same effect.

If you're having difficulties at work or at home, if there are unresolved issues around events from your past, or if you're going through a difficult time, these can show up in the shape of a bad dream. It's even been suggested that we dream about these difficult events, so that we can heal from them. When a person is experiencing post-traumatic stress for example, they may find sleep harder because they have nightmares of what happened; however, the research suggests that dreams may be part of the healing process.

According to Lisa LaBracio:

*Stress neurotransmitters in the brain are much less active during the REM stage of sleep, even during dreams of traumatic experiences, leading some researchers to theorise that one purpose of dreaming is to take the edge off painful experiences to allow for psychological healing.*[76]

Nightmares can make sure we take steps to acknowledge the "problem"; it's a bit like the volume going up – the music is so loud we have to do something about it. When the dream isn't being "heard", you might find it reoccurs until you seek an explanation. Nightmares can make us pay attention to what's really going on when we're ready.

Around the world, different cultures and traditions have ways of managing bad dreams; it's one of the reasons dreamcatchers exist. Looking for an explanation is another way, by exploring and deciphering the message – understanding what caused it, could stop it reoccurring. Talking to a professional can help take the fear out of addressing the dream itself. Sometimes nightmares appear far worse than their explanations actually are.

One lady told me about a dream she'd had, where an old-fashioned phone on the table was ringing. As she got closer, she saw the phone was covered in blood, and what looked like the guts of an animal. Although it kept ringing, she was frightened to pick up the phone. When I asked her if there was someone she needed to talk to but was putting it off, she said yes. There was a family member she needed to *pick up the phone* and talk to, but was afraid of doing it. After we had this conversation (and she made the phone call), she never had the dream again.

If you are worried about the cause or effect of your nightmares, particularly if they're affecting your sleep or mood, be sure to speak to your doctor as soon as possible. Lucid dreaming has been suggested as one technique which may help with nightmares in the right circumstances (more on this later too).

I described Old Hag Syndrome earlier, the feeling of a presence in the room; a common experience which feels like a nightmare. Often accompanied with a feeling of paralysis – that you can't move, or shout out (or if you do make a "strange" squealing sound), it can also be accompanied with a feeling of pressure on the chest. The paralysis should only last a few minutes but it does feel scary.

All of these can be a symptom of stress, or sleep deprivation, the many techniques including mindfulness are proven to help.

As confusing and even awful as dreams and nightmares might seem, they are important, and as we've seen a pathway to healing. We might not like them, but they usually have something important to say. Where a dream speaks, a nightmare shouts possibly until you pay attention, or the cause goes away.

*Nod to a Dream Movie: A dream within a dream – where you wake up, or think you have, then actually wake up – is sometimes known as a "false awakening", or "dream layer", which is loosely depicted in the 2010 movie* Inception *(Warner Bros). Children can have this dream just like adults, where they dream they've woken up and started their day (e.g. brushing their teeth), then actually wake up. Some researchers describe this as "pre-lucidity" because you may have some sense that something's not quite right about that reality. This type of dream may also be a sign you're overtired or may be a little stressed; this type of experience has also been reported when people are coming round from an anaesthetic. In the movie* Inception, *the layers were used to discover people's secrets or plant an idea in someone's mind whilst asleep. To date – and somewhat reassuringly – this hasn't been knowingly achieved in the scientific world.*

## Nightmare or Night Terror?

A nightmare is a bad dream that usually occurs during Rapid Eye Movement (REM) Sleep. During REM sleep, we are usually physically paralysed so that we can't carry out whatever we're dreaming. When the person wakes up, they can tell you the dream they had.

However, a night terror is where a person may thrash about or scream, and not recognise you when you speak or try to comfort them (because they're not fully awake). They are also likely to have little memory of it the next day. These are particularly common in children aged three to eight years old,[77] and for a small percentage, may continue in to adulthood. Overtiredness, anxiety, a full bladder or even a loud noise outside could be a cause.

## Lucid Dreaming

When you become aware that you're dreaming it's called a Lucid Dream.

It's a handy technique for resolving nightmares, for example, but it pays to know what you're doing and why. Where it can be helpful to change the ending of a dream, if say you dream you're being chased by a monster where it's a metaphor (you might say something is a "beast" of a problem) you can use lucid dreaming to turn and face your fear.

However, becoming lucid might not always be the best way to resolve the trauma of a real-life event that cannot be changed, and seeking professional help may be more useful; a technique like Eye Movement Desensitisation and Reprocessing (EMDR) may be a suitable alternative. EMDR is a psychotherapy treatment originally designed to alleviate the distress associated with traumatic memories, and connected to the biological mechanisms involved in REM sleep.[78]

Some people actively encourage lucid dreaming as a way to become "awake" in the dream, and use this "hybrid state of consciousness"[79] as an opportunity to practise a presentation at work or to see what it would be like to transport themselves into space. Charlie Morley, whose work around the shadow I mentioned earlier, has also written several books on the topic. In his book, Dreams of Awakening, he describes a "lucidity spectrum":

*Dreaming is not as clear-cut as just "lucid" or "non-lucid". There is rather, a lucidity spectrum based on the degrees of awareness within the dream, ranging from a suspicion that we might be dreaming to fully conscious reflective awareness.*

He goes on to explain four levels beginning with Pre-Lucid, a term coined by Celia Green, to "describe the state in which we critically question the reality of a dream." It's those moments in a dream when we might have a suspicion we're dreaming, because something's not quite right.

Semi-Lucid is, as Morley describes it, that "A-ha!" moment when you realise you might be dreaming, but then either slip back in to the dream, or wake yourself up.

Fully Lucid is when you're aware that you're dreaming and can start to influence the dreamscape. In this type of dream you're interacting with people and your surroundings as you would in waking reality, e.g. we can control our opening of a door, so that a cat can come in.

Finally, there is the Super-Lucid state, a term Morley borrowed from Robert Waggoner. In this dreaming state, instead of opening a door to let the cat in, we walk through the wall to join the cat in the garden. We move beyond the parameters of what seems real in the waking world, and can manipulate our surroundings to work for us.

An example of this may be when you become aware you're flying in a dream – not in an aeroplane, but as if you can actually fly. You know you cannot fly in real life, so as soon as you're flying in a dream, you might realise that you're dreaming.

In my flying dreams, I fly like Iron Man; I have invisible thrusters in my hands which control my speed and height. If I lean forward, I fly faster; if I lean back, I slow down. If I put my thrusters on, I go up; if I turn them off, I float back down. (Incidentally, over the years I've met many people who fly in their dreams, and each one has a slightly different way to another. Some fly like they're swimming, with breast stroke or front stroke, others similar to Superman, but without the cape.)

Regular lucid dreaming can take time and practice, so don't be disappointed if you don't have lucid dreams as often as you'd like or have tried to become lucid but have been unsuccessful.

You can also allow your mind to roam freely in dreams which of themselves can tackle problems and find answers too. Your dreams may be useful to you without telling them how you want them to end, but lucid dreaming can certainly help take charge of their content if you want to, and under proper instruction. Morley does do workshops (I have met him and he is an engaging and passionate speaker), and now because of the pandemic, I'm sure many will be online (www.charliemorley. com).

## Mutual Dreaming

I mentioned earlier the movie Inception (Warner Bros), in which Leonardo DiCaprio plays Dom Cobb – a fugitive who could infiltrate dreams in order to discover secrets. The film covered a number of different concepts, including the idea of a dream within a dream mentioned earlier, but also that two people can appear in each other's dream at the same time. So, can this happen? Apparently so.

Although undoubtedly more research will need to be done, it does appear possible that two people can have the same dream on the same night and each appear in another's dream. I say this because I've spoken with many people who have appeared in someone else's dream and vice versa – without any forward planning or conversations about dreams, only to discover the next day they were in the same time and place. Examples of this included two close work colleagues, a couple, a mother and daughter, and two best friends.

Some have tried to plan it, through the practice of Lucid Dreaming, but like any experiment the results can vary. In any event, and as with any Lucid Dreaming exercise, I would encourage you to make sure you feel safe with your dream partner, and if you are going to plan it, come to a mutual agreement on the arrangements, and only under the guidance of someone who knows what they're doing.

With those I spoke with, they were *not* aware they are dreaming at the time, it was only when they spoke of it, they realised they'd shared the same experience.

## Past Life Dreams

Sometimes you can have a dream which makes no sense because it's set in another time or place – one that you don't recognise –

and nothing about it reflects the life you're living now. I'm not talking about the time you dreamt you were in the house you used to live in as a child, or the school you used to go to when you were young (more on that under Anxiety Dreams); the ones I mean appear as if they're happening in a time before you were born.

Whilst the reasons we have this type of dream can vary, Jung postulated that we inherit the memory of human culture. This would explain why so many symbols appear across the globe, and can have similar interpretations. We could argue, if we inherit the memories of our ancestors, that it's possible a daughter for example could inherit her mother's memory at the point she was conceived.

One lady, I'll call her Tara, said one day she had a dream which appeared as if it was in the late sixties/early seventies, i.e. before she was born. In the dream she was wearing a beautiful dress above the knee, a bit like a smock, and her hair looked like Farrah Fawcett in the original *Charlie's Angels*. She said this dream made no sense to her as she recognised literally nothing about it, not even where she was, although it had a familiarity about it.

The next time she saw her mum, she described the dress and her surroundings, and how weird and yet strangely familiar the dream had felt. Her mum got up, went to an old family photo album, pulled out a picture and said, "Was this the dress?" There in the photo, was a picture of the mum, wearing what looked like the exact same dress and wearing her hair the way the daughter had in the dream. Was this a past life dream of a memory inherited from her mum? Or is it possible that she had seen that photo as a child and stored the memory for a later date? It's an area definitely worth more research.

One way people have said they can recognise a past life dream is if it contains anything which is remotely modern, it's probably not. So if you appear as a knight in shining armour riding a horse in to battle and your mobile phone goes off, it might be more a metaphor for how every day feels at work.

## Creative Dreams

This is one of my favourite explorations of dreams, where people have used their content to inform their work. Famous examples of this include Albert Einstein, who was said to have dreamt the theory of relativity, I mentioned Keith Richards earlier who apparently dreamt the riff to *(I Can't Get No) Satisfaction*, and Salvador Dalí who is believed to have used some of Freud's Interpretation of Dreams to inspire his artwork. If you've ever seen a Dalí painting, suddenly everything makes sense.

Mary Shelley dreamt the story of *Frankenstein*, Robert Louis Stevenson was said to have dreamt *Jekyll and Hyde* and Stephenie Meyer, author of *The Twilight Saga*, was said to have dreamt her books from start to finish in one night. What's even more interesting, so the story goes, is that the place where the books are set was one that apparently Stephenie had never visited in waking life. Yet how the scenery appears in the blockbuster films, that later made celebrities of Kristen Stewart and Robert Pattinson, was exactly as it appeared in her dream.

## Predictive Dreams

The idea that dreams can predict the future is fascinating and complex. Like most unexplained phenomena, it would be great if we could prove its existence simply with hard evidence under a controlled study. However, from those I've spoken with, you can't just decide that tonight you'll have a dream that will come true. Otherwise, we'd be asking for the lottery numbers every week.

Back in 1980 one newspaper did a study where 42 per cent of people felt they'd had at least one dream which then came true; whenever I've appeared on telly and the producers have done a poll the night before, the results are about the same. This certainly suggests predictive dreaming is more common than we might think.

The International Association for the Study of Dreams (IASD) acknowledges from research there are many impressive accounts from reliable sources which relate specifically to unlikely or unexpected events which have been dreamt about and then taken place. Those that have these types of dream often report that the dream itself simply "feels different".

But the idea that our dreams could predict what might happen next in our lives can be worrying; if we have a dream that someone we care about dies, we may naturally fear this is a prediction of things to come. So it helps to look at the different types of dreams which may fall in to this category.

*Precognitive Dreams:* are those where you may have had a thought prior to the dream which influenced the events which then happen or, as a result of the dream the thought became possible; in other words it was a forethought.

An example of this would be when you think about a meeting you have at work tomorrow, which you *know* is going to happen, and you dream about it the night before. The dream is predicting the future, but based on the fact you knew it would happen.

In the same way, you might dream of a friend's pregnancy or relationship breakdown before it happens, because of something they'd implicitly said on social media or conversations you'd been having which got your mind wondering. (Incidentally, pregnancy dreams can also be about giving birth to an idea, so if your friend turns out not to be pregnant, it might be that you will collaborate on a project together which, like pregnancy, needs to take time to grow.) Just as pregnancy dreams aren't always about having a baby, dreaming of someone's death doesn't mean it will come true.

If someone we love is at the end of their life and we know

their death is going to happen, we may dream about it; that would be classed as precognitive. In the same way a dream can help us rehearse a job interview, it can help prepare us on some level for the death of a loved one. This *doesn't* mean though that every time we dream about death it's going to come true. Whilst it acknowledges that death is part of life, it is also a metaphor for change and transformation. Death dreams can be a fear it might happen, rather than the reality itself. If you had a sense someone was seriously unwell and then they died, your dream *didn't* make it happen, just as if you dream someone dies, that *doesn't* mean they will.

This is the paradox of predictive dreams, you never know for sure unless it happens, so can only do what you can do; live every day as far as possible in a meaningful and healthy way.

*Prophetic Dreams:* Sometimes known as "Divine Dreams" because of references in religious texts, they are most famous in the context of a natural disaster or global event, which then comes true. A famous example of this would be those who reportedly cancelled their tickets aboard the *RMS Titanic* on the strength of the fact that they dreamt it would sink. Sometimes known as "Omen Dreams", again thankfully, just because you dream something, doesn't mean it's going to come true.

Those who dreamt the *Titanic* would sink, might have had a fear of sailing which manifested in their dreams, they could have cancelled their tickets on the strength of that alone. I've spoken to literally hundreds of people who dream something awful will happen, often involving travel – aeroplane and car crashes being the most popular (see *Anxiety Dreams*) – and nothing bad ever does.

*Prodromal (or prognostic):* Psychiatrist Dr Robin Royston suggested in an article, which appeared in *The Times* in 2004, that dreams can also highlight signs of illness within the body through their symbolised content and the language we use to describe them. So it's not that the dream is predicting anything as such, it's simply your mind bringing what is already happening in your body in to conscious awareness.

All this is not to say that there aren't some unexplained examples throughout history, so I've given food for thought to these too. In religious writings, stories of dreams which predicted the future are well known. In Buddhism, Maya, the Buddha's mother, had a dream which predicted, albeit through metaphor, who her son would become.

There are also some well recorded events throughout history, of people who dreamt about large-scale incidents – like the *Titanic* – which then came true. Whilst some of these as I've said may have been fears manifested in a dream, there are some, on a less global scale, that remain unexplained. An example of this would be a lady, I'll call her Aisling, who came to me after one of my workshops and told me a version of the following story.

In the eighties, Aisling was a young woman who, by her own admission, knew absolutely nothing about football. One night, for reasons she couldn't fathom, she dreamt about a famous football match that was due that weekend. In her dream, a "lowly" team that never won anything scored the winning goal. She told her father about her dream; he laughed and said that was never going to happen. Nevertheless, Aisling decided to go down to the bookmakers, and put £1 on the underdogs to win. (Her father apparently laughed at that too.) Anyway, long story short: the underdogs won, and Aisling cleaned up at the bookies.

I can't tell you why Aisling's dream came true and others don't; maybe she'd heard something that filtered in to her dream, or maybe it really was a dream come true.

However, if you're worried that your dreams might predict the future, please remember that if people were having dreams like this all the time, it would be classed as a fact and no one would question it. In all the years I've been doing this work, I do know Aisling's dream with this level of literal accuracy, without metaphor, is extremely rare.

## Is it possible to spot a predictive dream?

The short answer to this is no, the only way to know for sure if a dream predicts the future is if, like Aisling's, it did. However, some people have said:

- they simply "knew" their dream to be predictive.
- the dream appeared in sepia (the old black-and-white-style photograph). However, one reason we dream in black and white might be because it reflects our mood, or that there's not enough excitement or "colour" in our life.
- it's like watching a movie – this is called a "Witnessing Dream". This has also been reported when in the process of becoming lucid, or when experiencing a past life dream. So the experience doesn't necessarily mean it's going to come true.
- anecdotally, it was around the time of the full moon.

I've been really careful to say in all of this, that dreams are so often a reflection of our grief, or a *fear* of loss, that we should consider these in some depth before concluding it must be a prediction. It's why I'll explain shortly that dreaming of your partner cheating is more likely to be an anxiety – a fear of losing them – rather than a truth. A fear of anything, including our own death or someone we love, is enough to prompt a dream about it. If the fear of your dream coming true is creating anxiety, then talk to someone as soon as possible.

This leads me on to talk finally about Anxiety Dreams, before we come on to look at how we interpret them.

## Anxiety Dreams

These can often seem like a nightmare, and can leave the dreamer feeling edgy or uneasy the next day. The key to anxiety dreams is to also note their frequency and regularity. As I'll come on to explain, and a benefit of a dream diary, noticing when and where you have the dream can also give you insight as to why you've had it.

I've emphasised that there is no one-size-fits-all philosophy, so my intention below is to just give you some food for thought. The example Dream Record, which appears later, may help you explore your own dreams for yourself. You might find that once you understand why you're having it, it stops, or the mindfulness activities described earlier may help.

Here is a list of some anxiety dreams, but I've covered some which would also fit in this category (like losing teeth) earlier in the section on grief. Of course there are many more, but these are some common, reoccurring ones. Remember these dreams can represent how you feel, rather than how things actually are.

### Turning up somewhere naked

This can be a regular dream for young people, particularly dreaming that they're turning up for school or a new job with no clothes on. It's also a common dream amongst celebrities, particularly those who appear on TV and Radio, or those who stand up in front of others perhaps to give a presentation.

One of the reasons for this, it's been suggested, is that being naked is a metaphor for vulnerability, just as we are naked and vulnerable when we are born. For example appearing naked might acknowledge a secret that's been shared, or a fear of making a mistake, that leaves you feeling "exposed".

Another theory is that it can mean you're feeling under scrutiny, when we are naked we would naturally think all eyes are on us. This could be why some people dream they walk down the aisle naked or turn up for a job interview with no clothes on. One of the interesting things about the naked dream, is that people often realise that no one else seems to be bothered that they've showed up somewhere starkers. This can be a sign that the problem isn't as big as you might think it is, and no one really minds about something that's been bothering you.

## Being chased

*My recurring dream is that I'm out in the street, being chased by hundreds of people, I'm wearing a very short vest... and I can't pull the front down.*

This description above was recorded by Ernie Wise, the famous comedian in Dreamland's *Celebrity Book of Dreams*. I mentioned a similar dream earlier, and it's especially common for people who might need to confront something – i.e. there's no getting away from it. Whether you're the one who's doing the chasing, or you don't know who's chasing you, you might have a sense that something's catching up with you. You might also be trying to "catch up" on an important deadline, or you're running behind on something at work. It can also represent a fear of being caught (if you've done something you shouldn't) or you catching something – like coronavirus. (You'll notice in Ernie's dream that he also can't cover himself up, another type of "naked dream".)

Many people say when they're being chased it feels like they're walking or running through treacle; there may be a physiological reason for that.

When we're dreaming, we're essentially physically paralysed; the most common theory is that so you don't carry out what you're doing in the dream. So it could be that your brain is sending a message to your legs that you need to move, but your legs are sending a message back to the brain that they can't.

## Being back at school

This dream can often reflect a period of learning and has been common during the pandemic; people have said they've "learned" something about themselves since the outbreak began. It's also a naturally common dream for teachers and presenters. The most common dream like this I've heard is where the dreamer has turned up for an exam they didn't know was happening, or hadn't prepared for. This may be an acknowledgement that you're feeling unprepared, or are feeling as stressed today as you were when you were back at school.

## Missing a train or bus

Any form of public transport in a dream, whether it's a bus, plane or train, can be about social skills, and how we interact with others – it can also represent the "journey of life". This is why I mentioned earlier that travel disasters can be anxiety dreams (not predictive). When we say we've "missed the bus" we mean we've missed an opportunity, maybe at work, or a chance with someone we like. Waiting for a train, could be that we're waiting or relying on someone else to get us where we want to be. In the same way a car crash is a metaphor for something being a disaster but not in literal terms (see *Can't stop a car*, below).

## Can't stop a car

Cars in dreams can represent status, but if we put our foot on the brakes and nothing happens, this can suggest we're not feeling in control. In the same way, if you're not driving the car, it's worth noting who is, as that can sometimes give a clue to who you think is in charge of your life – or at least some decisions – right now.

Cars can also symbolise what motivates and inspires you – what "drives" you – in life. Perhaps recently you've been feeling "stuck" or "at a crossroads" as to which direction to take in your life.

People sometimes dream about different parts of the car – taking a back seat could be a metaphor for avoiding a decision or watching the world go by. The engine is what "drives" the car, so think about what gets your "motor running" – what motivates you and what's stopping you getting where you want to be. The boot or trunk of the car can be useful storage, but also where we tend to dump things we don't want. It can get cluttered and dirty. In these cases it might be time for a clear out of the things that are taking up too much space in your life, or room in your head. In the same way as a house dream, what's going on both inside and outside the car can reflect how you feel. So if for example the house or car is run-down or "beaten up", that might be how you're feeling right now. If in the dream you have to "put your foot down", that might mean you need to be firmer with someone in your waking life.

## Partner Cheating

Infidelity dreams are ones I get asked about a lot, because people worry that it might be a warning of something about to come true. So I've gone in to a bit of detail on this especially as it ties in with my theory that dreams can reflect our grief and fear of loss.

The first thing to maybe think about with infidelity dreams is who is having the affair. If you dream your partner is cheating you may be worrying that your intuition is trying to give you a heads up and that you need to keep an eye on your partner. However, it may be more likely a fear of history repeating itself if a previous relationship ended this way, especially if there's unfinished business with an ex.

If you're worried about your relationship, have a chat with your partner about any concerns that may be influencing your dreams. Speak to a third-party organisation if it helps establish boundaries or highlights any relationship fears and worries. No one – certainly not a professional – should tell you your partner is having an affair just based on the strength of a dream you have had.

If you dream you're the one cheating, in some cases it may be there is not enough excitement in your relationship and you're looking for ways to spice it up. That doesn't mean you're not happy, but you may worry things are going stale; your dream may suggest it's time to freshen things up. Don't be fooled though – I mentioned earlier that dreams of having sex with someone else are often more about connection, power and control, *not* sex.

So just as death dreams aren't always about an ending, infidelity dreams aren't always about cheating. Perhaps you are feeling cheated by someone, that's short-changed you in another part of your life. Maybe a job or something else wasn't what you thought it would be. If you put yourself down, lack confidence in yourself or worry you're not meeting your partner's needs you could have this dream. That doesn't mean it's true, just that you worry about it.

Fear of losing a partner through death or illness can also cause a dream of having an affair, and some people who've recently had a bereavement may experience this. The dream creates the message that you may see the illness or the death as the third person in the relationship, winning and taking them away from you.

*Toilet Dreams*
Whenever we need the toilet in a dream, the interpretation may depend on whether or not you needed the loo in "real" life (remember Granger, I spoke about earlier).

Sometimes dreams can be influenced by things "outside" the dream (like being thirsty or busting to go) and this filters in. It's a bit like hearing the doorbell in your dream, then realising when you wake up someone did actually call at the door. So if you found you needed the toilet when you woke up, this may have influenced your dream content.

There are other meanings though, especially where the toilet door is missing in the dream. This is a common theme: for some people both doors and walls can disappear, leaving them feeling exposed and everyone's watching them "go". This can be interpreted that at the time of the dream you may have put something "out in the open", a bit like the naked dream, or put yourself in a situation where you were open to the scrutiny of others, very much like the naked dream. If the toilets are dirty, this might reflect your thoughts about hygiene – especially in a global pandemic when public messaging is all about washing our hands – or it can also feel like you've been left with all the crap.

Toilet dreams can also suggest that you are finding it difficult to get any privacy; it may be in waking life, you keep being disturbed or interrupted, even when you want to spend a penny. It might also be that there's some stuff you need to get rid of, but you haven't found a safe space yet to do so.

## Struggling to Communicate

One final dream I wanted to include is where we try to communicate in a dream but can't. I mentioned earlier that sometimes we can have dreams where we make a strange squeaking sound, and this might be because we're having a dream where we're trying to call out. Another might be where we're trying to dial a number in a phone but it's just not working (remember also the dream with trouble picking up the phone). With the loosing teeth dream I mentioned earlier, sometimes people describe the teeth crumbling in to their mouth, others describe pulling out bunting or cotton wool.

All of these suggest a problem with communication; it doesn't mean that we don't articulate ourselves well, it might be that someone's just not listening when we try, so our efforts to talk don't get heard.

With all these dreams, and thousands of others I've not included here, the healing begins when we understand why we're having them, what they might mean and how we can use those insights to aid the journey.

So let's have a look at how we can work with them.

# How We Can Work with Our Dreams

## The Role of Symbols

Before we look at the "why" of a dream, a good place to start is looking at the symbols appearing in it. Everything that we remember from a dream can be relevant, so to understand what it means, it makes sense to look at what stood out the most.

The challenge we often have is that the stuff that features doesn't always connect at first glance because we tend to take it literally.

If you dream of a dragon, for example, you might wake up puzzled or scared, because dragons aren't real (at least not as far as we know). If though the dragon might symbolise your mother-in-law who you're due to see tomorrow, suddenly everything might click in to place. What felt like a nightmare, might be a reflection of how you feel about the visit.

Even if your mother-in-law isn't scary, your dream might just be giving you the heads up to prepare, something sometimes known as Primitive Instinct Rehearsal Theory, believed to help us practise our fight or flight skills.[80] In dreams, things often appear in metaphor with a symbol representing the message itself.

A symbol can be a letter, character, figure or mark to designate something with an associated meaning. Many people are taught symbols and their meanings growing up, without realising it. The ⏻ (power-off symbol), for example, indicates that using this button will disconnect power to a device. It's universally recognised, and although there is no wording on it that says "on/off", we just "know" what it means.

There will be many symbols culturally that you'll have grown up with, that influence how you feel and what you do. When I was a child, whenever my dad saw a magpie he'd say, "Good morning, Mr Magpie, how are you and your wife?" Like black cats, depending on how we feel about them, their appearance can change the mood of our day. Whenever I ask a group if they believe black cats represent good luck or bad to them, the room is usually divided half and half. Symbols then form part of our unconscious library, and dreams use them to communicate a message.

Dreams can be literal and metaphorical.

If I dream about a red traffic light, I might be receiving the wisdom that I need to stop or slow down. Where Freud might have argued that a tunnel represents the birth canal, sometimes a cigar is just a cigar.

If there's one thing I've said throughout this book, it's that everyone is different; what one dream means to one person may have a different meaning for someone else. It's one reason why this section is perhaps surprisingly so short, because you already have everything you need including your own personal symbol library to figure it out.

Here are some things to think about though, when exploring your dreams. I've also included a template for recording in your journal if it helps.

- Think about the timing of your dream: why this and why now? Is a dream about the past reflective of something that's happening in your life at the moment? Also think about when it started; if a recurring dream began two years ago, what happened then might have prompted you to keep dreaming what you do now. In the case of grief, it's common to dream about people or events around anniversaries, including marriage, birthdays and the date of the loss.
- Who is in it, and why them? I mentioned earlier that, generally speaking, people who appear in your dreams can be relevant to the characters in your waking reality. Where some dreamologists will focus on archetypes, or

suggest that sometimes someone who appears in your dream is actually a manifestation of yourself, I've often found that if you dream about a colleague at work, for example, it could well be a message about them. That's not to say that we don't project our fears or concerns in to characters who appear in our dreams; I mentioned earlier the monster catching up with us in a dream might be a manifestation of a fear, just as a baby that's crying in a dream might symbolise your basic needs aren't being met. So like I say, the key could be to focus on who is in the dream, and why them.

- Look for themes: are there patterns to your dreaming emerging? For example, do you keep seeing particular places, people or symbols? Do certain numbers or colours keep featuring in the dream? Think about why that might be. If you keep seeing the number three, is that significant; for example, is it someone's door number, a month (e.g. March), or something you associate with spiritually? Numerology can provide fascinating insights on why numbers might appear in dreams. A book like *Life by Numbers* by Elizabeth Barber describes "universal number attraction".

- How did the dream make you feel? Feelings can be confusing in dreams, because how we feel when they happen might not be how we feel when we wake. Where you might be happy in the dream, you might feel sad as you come to; this is especially the case when a person dreams about someone they have loved and lost. I mentioned earlier that sex in dreams can be about control, power or connection, and not necessarily in a sexual way. This is why you might have sex with someone in a dream you *never* would in real life. If you enjoyed it in the dream, but were repulsed when you woke up, the dream might symbolise a power play where someone wants to "get one over"; it could equally be a shared desire for something to succeed. Remember to ask for help if your dreams reflect a past trauma or difficulty you're going through.

- Consider the metaphor, is this literal or not? Think about the symbols and how they appear in your dream. The template next might also help, as can a game of word association; what do you think of when you visualise this symbol? A friend once told me about a dream she had when her baby was born, where her mum kept swaddling the baby in layers of blankets and placing her in front of the fire. My friend would literally wake up in a sweat thinking the baby was going to overheat. When I asked her if she felt the dream was a metaphor or literal, she said, "Oh, it's literal! My mum keeps wrapping her up in too much clothing, and I'm worried she's going to get too hot!" Remember also the lady earlier where in her dream she described she "couldn't pick up the phone". This was a metaphor for the fact she was finding it difficult to speak to someone in particular. So maybe ask yourself, what were you able or unable to do and what does this represent?

- How stressed are you? This is an important question and makes the point that what's going on for us during the day can play out in our dreams at night, especially if we're not giving our thoughts or worries a platform whilst we're awake; we call it "Day Residue". Following some of the tips I've described in this book, including the One Hour Rule and making relaxation a priority before bedtime, might help to manage the content of your dreams. In the same way, managing Day Residue can help: at least a couple of hours before you go to bed, ask yourself if anything is hanging over from the day. Is there something you need to talk about, or that's playing on your mind which might otherwise find its way in to your dreams?

- Ask for help. I've highlighted this throughout the book,

but I can't emphasise this enough. There are many specialists and agencies who can help with the range of topics I've explored in this book, and it's important that you focus on self-care and well-being, especially when working with troubling or worrying dreams. Make your sleep and holistic health a priority, and reach out to those who can help if you need.

## Keeping a Dream Diary

If you've been having recurring dreams for a while (whether it's days, months or years), keeping a dream diary can help you notice patterns developing; it's a great tool for understanding why you have dreams when you do, especially if your dream content has been troubling you. You may start to notice you have a particular dream the night before you have a specific meeting, the anniversary of an event, or the day after you see a certain person.

Here are some top tips for keeping a dream diary. You can start it before you go to bed if you want (e.g. by writing the date), or complete it first thing in the morning if you prefer. Because everyone is different, I can't guarantee specific results but it can certainly help.

## 1. Wind down before bed

Described earlier in The Sleep Cycle Repair Kit, avoid doing things like going on the computer or taking exercise in the hours leading up to bedtime and avoid drinking alcohol. Enjoy a nice warm bath and try listening to some calming music. In the hours before that, make sure you have, as far as possible, dealt with Day Residue – any thoughts or worries outstanding from the day.

## 2. Set your intention

Before you go to bed, if you want to remember your dreams,

set the intention to recall them; this can include writing the date in your dream diary (see template). If there's something in particular you'd like to dream about, or something you'd like to know, write that in your diary too. Keep it helpful and healthy.

## 3. Try a mindfulness meditation

When you're in bed, try one of the activities described earlier, like listening to the natural flow of your breathing, and give yourself permission to relax.

## 4. Keep pen and paper by your bed

All you need to record your dreams is pen and paper; if it's easier (and more practical if it's still dark when you wake up) use an old-fashioned Dictaphone if you have one (and as long as it won't wake anyone else up!). Try not to use your voice notes though, if the light from your phone might wake you up.

## 5. Lay still when you wake up

As you feel you're coming to, stay still for a moment and concentrate on what's going through your mind, and any elements of the dream you can remember. Write down as much as you can within the first few minutes of waking, almost as if you are writing a story. (If you don't write it down straight away, you'll probably find the dream soon disappears.) Draw pictures where it's hard to describe what things looked like.

## 6. Pay attention to the details

Note colours, environments, the weather – everything that comes to mind from your dream. In particular, notice how you are feeling when you wake up compared to how you were feeling in the dream, and use the tips I described earlier. Jot down the "characters" within the dream and whether or not you recognise them, or the person/people they represent. Notice if you were part of what was happening, or simply observing it.

Then think about how this translates to what's going on for you in your life at the moment. Good questions to ask yourself are: why this, why them, and why now?

## 7. Be patient

Don't worry if it's been a while since you remembered a dream; if your intention is to remember them, and your dreams have something to tell you, they'll be along in no time.

## Example Dream Record Template

Date: .... (you can use the night of the dream, or the day you wake, just be consistent each time)

Any influencing factors that might affect your dreams, e.g. what's happening in your life right now, food/drink consumed, what you watched on the TV.........

What and who appeared in the dream? What was the content? Include characters, scenery and symbols if they stand out and write as if telling a story if it helps..........

Look at the language: are there any metaphors or analogies?

Is there a theme to this dream, and is it reoccurring? For example, are you always in a particular place or with a particular person?

How did you feel in the dream? How do you feel now?

Thoughts on what this dream might mean.........

What helpful action could I take as a result of this dream?

## Before You Go To Sleep Tonight

1. Look in the mirror if you can. Remind yourself that you have a right to be here; that you belong. If you can, tell yourself how amazing you are, at the very least that you are enough. Celebrate the successes of today if you want, even the little things you've achieved, like getting up and washing your face. Find one tiny thing you feel you can appreciate about your day, like the socks that keep your feet warm, or the coffee that tasted just right.

2. When you get in to bed, and if it helps, focus on your breath; just notice that you're breathing right now. Don't worry whether it's fast or slow, or deep or shallow, just let the air flow freely. Take three deep breaths if you want to, remember you're in control. Then sink in to the natural rhythm of your breath. Place your hand over your heart or on your belly just to stay present in this moment. If it helps, repeat the words as many times as it helps, "May I be safe and free from fear. May I be happy and at ease."

3. If your mind wanders, remind yourself that a thought is just a thought. It doesn't need your time or your energy. The past and the future only exist as thoughts. And now is all there is.

And so, to bed.

# Useful Links

If you're worried about your physical or mental health, speak to your doctor as soon as possible. If you are in need of urgent medical assistance please call 999, or 111 if you're in the UK and concerned for your well-being.

This section contains some links for the UK which may be useful; if you're outside of the UK you may find equivalents in your area. This is not an exhaustive list, and a link doesn't mean the content is recommended, just that you may find it useful.

If you're struggling with your mental health, and need someone to talk to, remember **Samaritans**: are available 24/7 on 116 123 > http://Samaritans.org

You can also search **local Crisis Support** > www.nhs.uk/Service-Search/Crisis support/LocationSearch/329

**Victim Services during Coronavirus** > https://www.gov.uk/guidance/coronavirus-covid-19-victim-and-witness-services

Domestic Abuse: Government Guidance During Coronavirus> **https://www.gov.uk/guidance/domestic-abuse-how-to-get-help**

**Safety advice for survivors of domestic abuse during COVID-19** (Women's Aid) > https://www.womensaid.org.uk/covid-19-coronavirus-safety-advice-for-survivors/

**Talking to Young People about Coronavirus via Young Minds>** https://youngminds.org.uk/find-help/looking-after-yourself/

coronavirus-and-mental-health/

**Trouble Accessing Your GP**: Healthwatch > https://www.
healthwatch.co.uk/
"Visiting the doctor in difficult times" (article) >
https://helpingyousparkle.com/2019/06/18/visiting-your-
doctor-in-difficult-times/

**For latest public information on COVID-19** >
https://www.gov.uk/guidance/coronavirus-covid-19-
information-for-the-public

For **help with anxiety connected to hand hygiene** >
https://www.nhs.uk/conditions/obsessive-compulsive-
disorder-ocd/symptoms/ (NHS page on OCD)

**Mental Health**
If you're worried about a young person –
**Papyrus**: (preventing suicide in young people) 0800 068 41 41
https://www.papyrus-uk.org/help-advice
**Young Minds**: https://youngminds.org.uk/find-help/looking-
after-yourself/
Also:
**Powher** provide an advocacy service particularly around mental
health and work >
https://www.pohwer.net/
**Combat Stress** (UK Veterans Mental Health Charity):
http://combatstress.org.uk 0800 138 1619
**Mind** information leaflets on different types of mental health
condition:
http://mind.org.uk
**Heads Together** Tips for Talking: http://headstogether.org.uk/
tipsfortalking
**Autism Awareness** > https://www.autism.org.uk/

**Eating Disorders** – Beat Eating Disorders
> https://www.beateatingdisorders.org.uk/
Seasonal Affective Disorder: Mind Leaflet >
https://www.mind.org.uk/media-a/2952/sad-2019.pdf

**Pregnancy Mental Health**
**Maternity Action** is a UK charity committed to improving the
   health and well-being of pregnant women, partners and
   young children:
www.maternityaction.org.uk
**Refuge** – Information about Pregnancy and Domestic Abuse:
http://www.refuge.org.uk/get-help-now/
**TalkMum** – A community for Mums and Mums to Be >
www.talkmum.com/2012/05/coping-with-stress-during-
   pregnancy/ **Elaine Hanzak** is a speaker and author of two
   books around post-natal depression> http://hanzak.com
Raising awareness of post-natal depression **The Joanne
   (Joe) Bingley Memorial Foundation** > http://www.
   joebingleymemorialfoundation.org.uk
**Tommy's** Premature Baby Charity Tommy's > https://www.
   tommys.org/prematurity
Frequently Asked Questions:
https://pregnancymentalhealth.net/frequently-asked-
   questions/ (website by Delphi Ellis)
**NHS Choices** – pregnancy and mental health:
http://www.nhs.uk/Conditions/pregnancy-and-baby/pages/
   mental-health-problems-pregnant.aspx
**NHS Choices** – post-natal depression:
http://www.nhs.uk/Conditions/Postnataldepression/Pages/
   Introduction.aspx
**Mind information leaflet – Peri-natal Mental Health**:
http://www.mind.org.uk/information-support/types-of-
   mental-health-problems/postnatal-depression-and-
   perinatal-mental-health/

**Calm Zone** (specifically for men): https://www.thecalmzone. net/help/get-help/ https://pregnancymentalhealth.net/2016/10/21/ante-natal-and-post-natal-depression-and-anxiety-in-men/

**Financial or Legal** – Citizens Advice > https://www. citizensadvice.org.uk/

**Bereavement**

National Bereavement Partnership: The National Bereavement Partnership COVID-19 Hub provides a platform for associated practical advice services, support assistance and information to all those affected by the COVID-19 pandemic> https://www.nationalbereavementpartnership.org/

At a Loss > https://www.ataloss.org/

Cruse Bereavement Care > http://cruse.org.uk

National Bereavement Service includes guides on Registering a Death and Coroner's Inquests > https://www.nationalbereavementservice.org/about

Chums (for children) > chums.uk.com/

Dying Matters > https://www.dyingmatters.org/

Child Bereavement UK > https://childbereavementuk.org/

SOBS (for those bereaved by suicide) > https://uksobs.org/

The Compassionate Friends (Death of a Child) > https://www. tcf.org.uk

The Way Foundation (Death of a partner under 51 years of age) https://www.widowedandyoung.org.uk

Stillbirth and Neonatal Death Society > sands.org.uk/sands-here-support-you

Miscarriage Association > https://www.miscarriageassociation. org.uk/

National Homicide Service (Bereaved Families affected by Homicide) > https://www.victimsupport.org.uk/more-us/why-choose-us/

specialist-services/homicide-service

21 Things You Might Need to Do When Someone Dies (UK Care Guide) > https://ukcareguide.co.uk/dealing-with-bereavement/

Blue Cross Pet Bereavement > https://www.bluecross.org.uk/pet-bereavement-and-pet-loss

**Domestic Abuse**

Refuge > www.refuge.org.uk/

Respect UK > https://www.respect.uk.net

National Domestic Abuse Helpline: 0808 2000 247 > https://www.nationaldahelpline.org.uk

LGBT DA Helpline https://www.womensaid.org.uk/the-survivors-handbook/lgbt/

**Survivors of Rape and Sexual Assault**

Rape Crisis UK > https://rapecrisis.org.uk/

Survivors UK – Male Rape and Abuse > https://www.survivorsuk.org/ways-we-can-help/online-helpline/

Male Survivors Helpline > https://www.safeline.org.uk/national-mens-abuse-helpline-is-launched/

Relationship counselling > www.relate.org.uk

**Managing Addiction**

Drug addiction > https://www.nhs.uk/live-well/healthy-body/drug-addiction-getting-help/

Find alcohol addiction services > https://www.nhs.uk/service-search/other-services/Alcohol%20addiction/LocationSearch/1805

Quit Smoking > https://www.nhs.uk/better-health/quit-smoking/

# Endnotes

1. https://www.nationalgeographic.com/science/2020/04/coronavirus-pandemic-is-giving-people-vivid-unusual-dreams-here-is-why/
2. https://news.sky.com/story/health-study-finds-brits-are-the-worst-sleepers-10635198
3. Big Sleep Report, Dr Guy Meadows (2017)
4. Referenced in the Big Sleep Report, Bensons for Beds (2017).
5. https://globalnews.ca/news/2054861/why-the-who-is-warning-about-poor-sleep-and-heart-health (30/12/18)
6. https://www.newscientist.com/article/mg23731700-200-why-dreaming-is-vital-unlocking-the-power-of-rem-sleep (2/1/19)
7. https://med.stanford.edu/news/all-news/2020/06/william-dement-giant-in-field-of-sleep-medicine-dies-at-91.html
8. http://news.bbc.co.uk/1/hi/health/4228707.stm
9. Big Sleep Report, Meadows (2017)
10. As of August 2020.
11. *The Sleep Revolution*, Huffington, A. (WHAllen, 2016)
12. https://www.psychologytoday.com/ie/blog/between-the-lines/201905/whats-making-so-many-young-people-depressed (10/8/19)
13. https://sleepcouncil.org.uk/first-ever-great-british-bedtime-report/ (2013)
14. The Great British Sleep Survey (2012)
15. https://edition.cnn.com/2015/10/29/health/sleep-like-your-ancestors/index.html (2017)
16. https://www.ncbi.nlm.nih.gov/pmc/articles/PMC2128646/ (2007)
17. https://www.sleepfoundation.org/articles/teens-and-sleep
18. https://www.independent.co.uk/life-style/orthosomnia-sleep-disorder-insomnia-restless-fitness-trackers-

fitbit-a8278391.html (2018)
19. https://www.verywellmind.com/how-to-cope-with-fomo-4174664 (2020)
20. https://www.bupa.co.uk/newsroom/ourviews/nine-benefits-good-night-sleep
21. https://abcnews.go.com/Health/extreme-sleep-deprivation-navy-seals-handle-sleep/story?id=35286158 (2015)
22. https://www.open.edu/openlearn/history-the-arts/history/history-science-technology-and-medicine/history-technology/the-industrial-revolution-and-time
23. http://www.historyofwatch.com/clock-inventors/who-invented-clock/
24. https://en.wikipedia.org/wiki/Eight-hour_day
25. https://yougov.co.uk/topics/economy/articles-reports/2018/08/15/majority-employees-check-work-emails-while-holiday
26. https://psychcentral.com/blog/your-brain-is-not-a-computer/ (2018)
27. Big Sleep Report, Meadows (2017)
28. https://www.mentalhealth.org.uk/news/mental-health-foundation-launches-im-fine-campaign (2016)
29. https://www.healthline.com/health-news/did-we-inherit-sleep-patterns-from-prehistoric-ancestors#1 (2017)
30. https://youtu.be/dqONk48l5vY What would happen if you didn't sleep? - Claudia Aguirre
31. https://www.ted.com/talks/rives_on_4_a_m?language=en Ted Talk 2007, Rives: The 4am Mystery
32. https://www.powerofpositivity.com/if-you-wake-up-at-the-same-time-every-night-this-may-be-why/ (2018)
33. https://www.bustle.com/p/why-do-scary-movies-cause-nightmares-experts-explain-the-relation-19216887 (2019)
34. https://www.mind.org.uk/information-support/types-of-mental-health-problems/seasonal-affective-disorder-sad/ (31/12/18)

35. https://medium.com/the-mission/this-is-why-you-are-addicted-to-your-thoughts-without-knowing-it-1aaa557784bd
36. https://www.mind.org.uk/information-support/types-of-mental-health-problems/obsessive-compulsive-disorder-ocd/about-ocd/
37. https://www.youtube.com/watch?v=sMsUGB_KV7s (2012)
38. *A Monk's Guide To Happiness*, Thubten, G. (Yellow Kite, 2019, p. 28)
39. http://lifedeathwhatever.com (2019)
40. https://www.gov.uk/government/publications/end-of-life-care-profiles-february-2018-update/statistical-commentary-end-of-life-care-profiles-february-2018-update (February 2018)
41. https://www.which.co.uk/news/2018/12/half-of-adults-dont-have-wills-but-what-happens-to-your-children-when-you-die/ (2018)
42. https://www.bbc.co.uk/news/stories-53267505 (2020)
43. https://www.ted.com/talks/nora_mcinerny_we_don_t_move_on_from_grief_we_move_forward_with_it?language=en (2018)
44. https://whatsyourgrief.com/64-examples-of-disenfranchised-grief/ (2018)
45. https://www.joincake.com/blog/inhibited-grief/ (2020)
46. https://www.researchgate.net/publication/230669310_Meaning_Reconstruction_in_the_First_Two_Years_of_Bereavement_The_Role_of_Sense-Making_and_Benefit-Finding
47. https://www.britishmuseum.org/collection/object/Y_EA10683-3 (2020)
48. https://ancientegypt.fandom.com/wiki/Papyrus_Chester_Beatty_3 (2020)
49. https://www.mariecurie.org.uk/blog/the-story-behind-the-yellow-hearts-in-windows/276536 (July 2020)

50. Derk-Jan Dijk and Raphaëlle Winsky-Sommerer (*New Scientist*, 4 February 2012)
51. https://www.sleepfoundation.org/articles/connection-between-sleep-and-overeating (2020)
52. https://www.ted.com/talks/judson_brewer_a_simple_way_to_break_a_bad_habit (November 2015)
53. https://youtu.be/AdKUJxjn-R8 "Forget Big Change, Start with a Tiny Habit" (December 2012)
54. Catherine de Lange, How to Nap Like a Pro (*New Scientist* article, 25 May 2016)
55. https://www.sciencedaily.com/releases/2017/06/170605085326.htm (2017)
56. https://aasm.org/delayed-sleep-phase-syndrome-linked-to-irregular-menstrual-cycles-premenstrual-symptoms-in-women/ (American Academy of Sleep Medicine)
57. https://www.stylist.co.uk/life/sunday-night-time-anxiety-stress-sophrology-techniques-reduce-monday-worry/345190 (2020)
58. https://www.mindful.org/bottled-up-emotions-at-work-lead-to-burnout/ (2018)
59. https://www.cell.com/current-biology/fulltext/S0960-9822(16)30174-9
60. *The Voices Within*, Fernyhough, C. (Wellcome Collection, 2017, pp. 3, 10)
61. https://www.bbc.co.uk/news/magazine-17105759 (2012)
62. https://www.rsph.org.uk/our-work/policy/wellbeing/sleep.html (2016)
63. https://sleepcouncil.org.uk/advice-support/sleep-advice/perfect-sleep-environment/ (2020)
64. https://www.psychologytoday.com/gb/blog/the-right-mindset/202004/the-90-second-rule-builds-self-control (2020)
65. https://www.getselfhelp.co.uk/stopp.htm
66. Adapted from *The Little Book of Affirmations*, by Ani Trime.

67. https://theconversation.com/the-science-of-sleep-how-sharing-your-dreams-could-help-to-improve-your-relationships-137193 (2020)
68. https://www.newscientist.com/article/dn22205-location-of-the-mind-remains-a-mystery/#ixzz6ZMXx2mH9 (August 2012)
69. *Learn to Dream*, Fontana, D. (DBP, 1996)
70. https://www.rockefeller.edu/news/17839-jonathan-winson-dies-at-84/ (2008)
71. http://www.mythfolklore.net/3043mythfolklore/reading/rumi/pages/01.htm
72. https://dreamstudies.org/tag/carl-jung/
73. *New Scientist*, No 3187 (July 2018)
74. *Dreaming Through Darkness*, Morley, C. (Hay House, 2017)
75. *Nightmare*, Shulman, S. (David and Charles, 1979)
76. https://blog.ed.ted.com/2016/01/25/why-do-we-dream-7-theories-from-science-in-ted-ed-gifs/ (2016)
77. https://www.nhs.uk/conditions/night-terrors/
78. https://www.emdr.com/what-is-emdr/
79. *Dreams of Awakening*, Morley, C. (Hay House, 2013)
80. https://blog.ed.ted.com/2016/01/25/why-do-we-dream-7-theories-from-science-in-ted-ed-gifs/ (2016)

# Author Bio

Delphi is a qualified counsellor, well-being trainer and mindfulness practitioner who has worked in a therapeutic setting since 2002. She started her helping career supporting people in grief, mainly those bereaved by murder and suicide. She now works in the community promoting mental health maintenance and recovery, mindful leadership and workplace wellness, with clients in both 1-1 and group settings. She offers practical insights aimed at helping you find your mojo and getting your sparkle back. Delphi is asked to appear regularly on TV and radio talking about dreams, with appearances on ITV's *This Morning*, *Loose Women* and presented the Guide to Sleep on *Daybreak*.

www.DelphiEllis.com
AnswersInTheDark.com

# Recent bestsellers from O-Books are:

## Heart of Tantric Sex
Diana Richardson
Revealing Eastern secrets of deep love and intimacy to Western couples.
Paperback: 978-1-90381-637-0 ebook: 978-1-84694-637-0

## Crystal Prescriptions
The A-Z guide to over 1,200 symptoms and their healing crystals
Judy Hall
The first in the popular series of eight books, this handy little guide is packed as tight as a pill-bottle with crystal remedies for ailments.
Paperback: 978-1-90504-740-6 ebook: 978-1-84694-629-5

## Take Me To Truth
Undoing the Ego
Nouk Sanchez, Tomas Vieira
The best-selling step-by-step book on shedding the Ego, using the teachings of *A Course In Miracles*.
Paperback: 978-1-84694-050-7 ebook: 978-1-84694-654-7

## The 7 Myths about Love...Actually!
The Journey from your HEAD to the HEART of your SOUL
Mike George
Smashes all the myths about LOVE.
Paperback: 978-1-84694-288-4 ebook: 978-1-84694-682-0

## The Holy Spirit's Interpretation of the New Testament
A Course in Understanding and Acceptance
Regina Dawn Akers
Following on from the strength of *A Course In Miracles*, NTI
teaches us how to experience the love and oneness of God.
Paperback: 978-1-84694-085-9 ebook: 978-1-78099-083-5

## The Message of A Course In Miracles
A translation of the Text in plain language
Elizabeth A. Cronkhite
A translation of *A Course in Miracles* into plain, everyday
language for anyone seeking inner peace. The companion
volume, *Practicing A Course In Miracles*, offers practical lessons
and mentoring.
Paperback: 978-1-84694-319-5 ebook: 978-1-84694-642-4

## Your Simple Path
Find Happiness in every step
Ian Tucker
A guide to helping us reconnect with what is really important in
our lives.
Paperback: 978-1-78279-349-6 ebook: 978-1-78279-348-9

## 365 Days of Wisdom
Daily Messages To Inspire You Through The Year
Dadi Janki
Daily messages which cool the mind, warm the heart and guide
you along your journey.
Paperback: 978-1-84694-863-3 ebook: 978-1-84694-864-0

## Body of Wisdom
Women's Spiritual Power and How it Serves
Hilary Hart
Bringing together the dreams and experiences of women across
the world with today's most visionary spiritual teachers.
Paperback: 978-1-78099-696-7 ebook: 978-1-78099-695-0

## Dying to Be Free
From Enforced Secrecy to Near Death to True Transformation
Hannah Robinson
After an unexpected accident and near-death experience, Hannah
Robinson found herself radically transforming her life, while a
remarkable new insight altered her relationship with her father, a
practising Catholic priest.
Paperback: 978-1-78535-254-6 ebook: 978-1-78535-255-3

## The Ecology of the Soul
A Manual of Peace, Power and Personal Growth for Real People
in the Real World
Aidan Walker
Balance your own inner Ecology of the Soul to regain your
natural state of peace, power and wellbeing.
Paperback: 978-1-78279-850-7 ebook: 978-1-78279-849-1

## Not I, Not other than I
The Life and Teachings of Russel Williams
Steve Taylor, Russel Williams
The miraculous life and inspiring teachings of one of the World's
greatest living Sages.
Paperback: 978-1-78279-729-6 ebook: 978-1-78279-728-9

## On the Other Side of Love
A woman's unconventional journey towards wisdom
Muriel Maufroy
When life has lost all meaning, what do you do?
Paperback: 978-1-78535-281-2 ebook: 978-1-78535-282-9


## Practicing A Course In Miracles
A translation of the Workbook in plain language, with
mentor's notes
Elizabeth A. Cronkhite
The practical second and third volumes of The Plain-Language
*A Course In Miracles*.
Paperback: 978-1-84694-403-1 ebook: 978-1-78099-072-9


## Quantum Bliss
The Quantum Mechanics of Happiness, Abundance, and Health
George S. Mentz
*Quantum Bliss* is the breakthrough summary of success and
spirituality secrets that customers have been waiting for.
Paperback: 978-1-78535-203-4 ebook: 978-1-78535-204-1


## The Upside Down Mountain
Mags MacKean
A must-read for anyone weary of chasing success and happiness
– one woman's inspirational journey swapping the uphill slog for
the downhill slope.
Paperback: 978-1-78535-171-6 ebook: 978-1-78535-172-3

**Your Personal Tuning Fork**
The Endocrine System
Deborah Bates
Discover your body's health secret, the endocrine system, and
'twang' your way to sustainable health!
Paperback: 978-1-84694-503-8 ebook: 978-1-78099-697-4


Readers of ebooks can buy or view any of these bestsellers by
clicking on the live link in the title. Most titles are published
in paperback and as an ebook. Paperbacks are available in
traditional bookshops. Both print and ebook formats are
available online.
Find more titles and sign up to our readers' newsletter at
http://www.johnhuntpublishing.com/mind-body-spirit
Follow us on Facebook at https://www.facebook.com/OBooks/
and Twitter at https://twitter.com/obooks